Th

MW01062261

"Zam is funny, smart and one hell of an educator. I commend her for sharing her own experience and writing a book about pleasure for women. All women need a Pleasure Plan."

—**Betty Dodson, PhD,** sexologist, Netflix sex educator, bestselling author of *Sex for One*

"Laura Zam's work is passionate, witty, psychologically astute, and filled with wisdom and good healing karma."

—**Susan Shapiro,** *New York Times* bestselling author of *Unhooked* and *Five Men Who Broke My Heart*

"In each of us, there is a quiet, bright voice, insisting on a life of pleasure and aliveness. This is the voice Laura uses to write this book — along with some wicked humor."

—**LiYana Silver,** coach and author of *Feminine Genius: The Provocative Path to Waking Up and Turning On the Wisdom of Being a Woman*

"Laura's healing is beautifully woven together in this memoir using humor and wit. So many people need to read this book to increase sex education, awareness, and hope for more pleasure in their life."

—**Rachel S. Rubin, MD,** urologist, sexual medicine specialist, and national health advocate

"Reading *The Pleasure Plan* feels like going on the ride with Zam and exiting the off-ramp wiser, much more hopeful, and, above all, more human."

—**Rosalyn Dischiavo,** author of *The Deep Yes: The Lost Art of True Receiving,* founder of Institute for Sexuality Education & Enlightenment

"An empowering journey helping women navigate their bodies, their bedrooms, and their health. Gorgeously told."

—**Nina Lorez Collins,** author of
*What Would Virginia Woolf Do? And Other Questions I Ask Myself
as I Attempt to Age Without Apology,* founder of The Woolfer

"God Bless Laura Zam for having the courage and sticktoitiveness to not only discover her own pathway to both healing and pleasure, but to provide a blueprint for us all to do the same."

—**Steph Jagger,** bestselling author of *Unbound: A Story of Snow
And Self-Discovery* and co-creator of Sacred Rebellion

"The Pleasure Plan is a fiercely empowering tale, an intimate portrait of a couple that is also a map for greater enjoyment of sex and connection. This is a book for all who seek sensual healing. Brave and inspiring!"

—**Aspen Matis,** bestselling author of *Girl in the Woods* and
Your Blue Is Not My Blue: A Missing Person Memoir

"A useful guide for people of all genders navigating complexities of the bedroom. Great for partners too. Funny, moving, and filled with tips!"

—**Robert Festinger,** screenwriter,
Academy Award nominee, *In the Bedroom*

"I'm so glad Laura didn't listen to her mother's advice: don't go for passion. In her witty, wide-ranging and wildly helpful book, she bravely reveals her healing journey for searingly painful issues that many barely acknowledge. Laura leads the way in forging a path for sexual healing. Pleasure Plan is an inspirational and pragmatic life-changer."

—**Bridgit Dengel Gaspard,** author of *The Final 8th:
Enlist Your Inner Selves to Accomplish Your Goals*

The Pleasure Plan

One Woman's Search for Sexual Healing

Laura Zam

Health Communications, Inc.
Boca Raton, Florida

www.hcibooks.com

To protect the privacy of individuals featured in this book, I have changed most names and identifying details. The exception applies to those who gave me explicit permission to present them without masking: Kurt, my husband; Shirley Serotsky and Ari Roth, who commissioned my one-person play; Diana and Richard Daffner, who run Intimacy Retreats; Betty Dodson and Carlin Ross, who run Bodysex Workshops; and Regena Thomashauer, who goes by Mama Gena. All dialogue and events are as I remember them. In a few places, I have altered chronology for better narrative flow.

**Library of Congress Cataloging-in-Publication Data
is available through the Library of Congress**

© 2020 Laura Zam

ISBN-13: 978-0-7573-2350-8 (Paperback)
ISBN-10: 0-7573-2350-2 (Paperback)
ISBN-13: 978-0-7573-2351-5 (ePub)
ISBN-10: 0-7573-2351-0 (ePub)

Pleasure epigraph printed by permission. From *Merriam-Webster.com* © 2019 by Merriam-Webster, Inc., *https://www.merriam-webster.com/dictionary/pleasure*.

All rights reserved. Printed in the United States of America. No part of this publication may be reproduced, stored in a retrieval system, or transmitted in any form or by any means, electronic, mechanical, photocopying, recording, or otherwise, without the written permission of the publisher.

HCI, its logos, and marks are trademarks of Health Communications, Inc.

Publisher: Health Communications, Inc.
      1700 NW 2nd Avenue
      Boca Raton, FL 33432-1653

Cover design by Larissa Hise Henoch
Interior design and formatting by Lawna Patterson Oldfield

For Kurt, Forever.

Pleasure

noun

1: DESIRE, INCLINATION

2: a state of gratification

3: sensual gratification . . .

4: a source of delight or joy

—Merriam-Webster

Contents

Author's Note

Dear Reader,

I am happy to meet you. I wrote *The Pleasure Plan* because my life expanded in so many ways because of my sexual healing journey. Instead of feeling embarrassment over my sex problems, I found bliss and a sense of power, which carried over into other areas of my life. Inspired by what I had discovered, and eager to help others, I became a sexuality educator. I also formalized my trauma education by becoming a Certified Trauma Professional.

Along with my personal narrative, I've included some self-help tips plus a resource section at the end of the book called "How to Create Your Own Pleasure Plan." These tips are designed for people of any gender identity, gender expression, sexual orientation, biological sex, and commitment style.

Here's to your pleasure!

Acknowledgments

It is with great pleasure that I acknowledge all the people who have helped make this book possible. I'll try to include everyone, but if I've interacted with you in the last couple of years, trust me, you have somehow contributed to this consuming, exhilarating project. My first order of gratitude goes to Ari Roth and Shirley Serotsky, formerly of Theater J, for commissioning the play *Married Sex*. I can't thank both of you enough for letting me write about my taboo sex problems, and for supporting my efforts to heal in this unique way. Also, a huge hug to Theater J staff and to Batya E. Feldman, who played a crucial role in getting my play to finally work. While on the subject of originating forces, I am deeply grateful to Susan Shapiro, literary dream maker extraordinaire. Sue, this book would not exist without your mentorship, guidance, and heart. Thanks also to Daniel Jones for publishing my essay "Healing Sought (Bring Your Own Magic)" in the *New York Times, Modern Love*. That essay opened many doors for me, changing the course of my life. Along similar lines, thank you Sarah Hepola for publishing a related essay, "How I Cured My *Sexual Dysfunction* Without a Pill" in *Salon*.

I am forever grateful to my amazing agent Laura Yorke. Laura, thank you for taking a chance on me, and for fighting so hard to get this book published. You are the warm, funny, fierce, wise agent I also wanted. I can't believe how lucky I am to be in your nurturing orbit, and to work with you. And speaking of luck, I am forever grateful to HCI Books for being so enthusiastic about this book from the get-go. Thank you Allison Janse, my amazingly talented editor, who has patiently put up with my neuroses, and who has given me so much space to organically grow this project. I am thankful for all your help shaping this book—and this author. Big, big thanks to other leadership and staff at HCI, particularly my savvy, fabulous HCI publicist, Kim Weiss. Thank you Larissa Hise Henoch for the perfect cover design, and Lawna Patterson Oldfield for gorgeous internal design. Thank you Simon & Schuster staff for your part in bringing this book into the hands of readers.

I would like to acknowledge the incredible developmental editors that helped me during different stages of this process: Nicole Bokat, Kimmi Auerbach Berlin, Beth Rashbaum, and Melissa Scholes Young. Individually, and collectively, you all taught me so much about writing. This book would not exist without your counsel and input. A special bow of gratitude goes to Jill Rothenberg, whose ideas and generosity got this project initially off the ground.

A huge debt is owed to all the people that served as early, and ongoing, readers for this memoir. In no particular order: Jamie Holland Hull, Julia Hager Tagliere, Frannie Hochberg-Giuffrida, Swati Khurana, Kelly O'Neal, Debra Perlson-Mishalove, Laura Ivers, Stephanie Donne, and the women of Writers and Critters. Love and appreciation to Julie Chibarro, who has given me the courage to pursue my artistic potential for the past twenty-six years. Julie, you are my rock, and the person I most look up to. This book would not have been possible without my Tuesday Night Salon: Ida Bostian, Vonetta Young, Tanya Senanayake, Joanna Urban, Anne Pellicciotto, Amy E. Allen, Beth Johnston, Sallie Crosby Hess, Di Jayawickrema, Christine Evans, Cassandra Marie Osvatics, Meeta Kaur, Lorine Kritzer Pergament, Leslie Pietrzyk, and others. A big hug to Neroli Lacey for recommending structure books, thinking about my story off-hours (with texts!), and for stepping in to be co-host—and friend—when I really needed it. Gratitude goes to West End Writers not already named: Cathy Alter, Lisa Leibow, and Lisa Friedman. A special shout-out to DMV Women Writers, especially Susan Keselenko Coll and Mary Kay Zuravieff, who've been supportive in critical ways. *The Pleasure Plan* owes its existence to dear friends who cheered me on throughout: Betsy Reinstein Dewy, Cheryl Hurwitz, Holly Segal, Allison Yorra, Susan Levin, Valerie Graff, Denise Woods, Maryanne Pollack, Molly McCloskey, and too many others to name. Thank you to Martin, Debbie, Chelsea, Jillian, and Sam, for letting me write about "The Zams." I'd like to thank Heather Schroder for reading early pages and offering very helpful feedback. Thank you, Nina Lorez Collins, for your generosity and support. Thank you, Jesse Klausmeier, for helping me better conceptualize the self-help portion of my book.

I am forever indebted to all the practitioners I saw during the period of time covered in this book. Wacky as this project was at times, each of these individuals offered me an essential, healing puzzle piece. Extra thanks to Carlin Ross, Betty Dodson, Nita Apple, Regena Thomashauer, Diana Daffner, Emily Nagoski, and Richard Daffner for reading chapter drafts and encouraging this project.

Thank you, Simone Nemes, for fab illustrations. And tremendous gratitude goes to Rachel Rubin, MD, for making sure I got the medical information right. I tip my hat to Robin Diamond for helping me fit this book into "the ecosystem," and for being such a brilliant ally. Tremendous thanks goes to Roz Dischiavo, founder of Institute for Sexuality Education and Enlightenment (ISEE), for her input on the Tips sections of this book, and for turning me into a sexuality educator. The writing of this book was partially funded by the DC Commission on the Arts and Humanities, through an Arts and Humanities Fellowship. I'd like to formally acknowledge their role and assistance. Thank you also to Brett Bevell for his part in my Hermitage Artist Residency at Omega Institute, where I worked on an early concept of this book.

Finally, thank you, Kurt, for allowing me to write about us, and for putting up with my crazy writing schedule. Mostly, though, thank you for finding me on Match.com. You are my life.

Prologue

Every Hooha Hang-Up in the DSM

August 2011

"**M**aybe you're just *not* a very sexual person," says Dr. Fay in a slow Southern drawl. I have come to this office to save my new marriage. After thirty years of searching, I've found a man I love who loves me back—at forty-eight. I never had reciprocity before, meaning a real relationship. But now I do. With Kurt, my miracle husband.

Kurt doesn't know the extent of my damage.

"What if I'm just broken?" I ask, my voice a shaky vibrato. I have never talked openly about the problems plaguing me since I was seventeen: low libido, orgasm challenges, and pelvic pain. I always assumed my obstacles were permanent. Is that true? "If my sexuality is broken," I venture, sitting taller on the maroon leather couch I'm sticking to, "I can fix it. Can't I?"

"Not if you have no libido," says Dr. Fay, an attractive marriage and family therapist specializing in hypnosis. "Look, it's fine to have no libido. You know that, right?"

I nod, thinking of grandmas, and nuns, and those that make *asexual* a lifestyle. But Fay's outfit—strange for a mental health professional, especially one who's middle-aged—puts notions in my head. A question pulls like thread from her gold metallic miniskirt. It sheds from her short-sleeved mohair sweater. She looks like an unwashed lover might come by right after I leave here. So I ask: "Can Eros be taught?"

The hypnotist chuckles, assuming I'm joking. I'm not. She tucks brown hair behind her ears and widens her pale green eyes. We have the same coloring, except I'm obviously nothing like her. "Would you like to hear about others in your situation?" she inquires. Without waiting for a response, she stands and begins pacing. "Now one client, she'd rather be waterboarded than sleep with *her* husband."

I know I should interrupt, revealing what I haven't shared yet—the experiment. Two weeks ago I implemented a strategy to finally heal, after thirty years. It started with no longer believing that pleasure is out of reach, or that it's dangerous. *To hell with fragility.* More feeling than fact, it seems like if I pressed on a thigh or clavicle, I could dislodge something, puncturing a vital organ.

Loneliness has done this to me.

I think of Kurt, and one night in particular. It was a summer evening, weeks after we met, and he was pushing me on a swing. Within seconds, I was up in the trees, all because of his force. *Not bad for fifty-one.* I let this overall impression of him—capable arms, uplifted cheeks when we'd stumbled upon the playground, our instantaneous agreement I must go on the swing—replace my imagined breakability. *He's incredible*, I thought, up in the sky and coming back down. A million neurons fired while I squealed, "Harder. Push harder."

As Dr. Fay regales me with tales of lacking lust, I force myself to think about why my bedroom is nothing like the swing. I *know* the reason, and she does too. I need to get this visit back on track. "I understand what you're telling me," I say in the middle of another depressing story. "But do you think we can talk about my trauma?"

I watch her hands find their way to her hips. Her pose makes me think she's forgotten what I disclosed in our previous telephone intake.

"That happened a loooong time ago," she says finally with a wave of pink manicure.

"I think it's related," I insist because *how could my issues not be related to trauma?* I explain that every therapist I've seen—six of them, spread out over geography and time—agreed there's a connection. My carnal health is surely tangled up in these sheets.

Silently, Dr. Fay strolls back to her purple velvet chair, which she commands like a throne. She crosses her toned bare legs and peers at me.

What if she's right about my past? These events *did* happen a long time ago. As for my therapists of yore, childhood was all they dwelled upon. Never what I should do with grown-up maladies I was left with, or how to improve mechanics, or how to navigate my pain. Not one shrink had knowledge of my full array of conditions. Even my gynecologist was stumped. Since I started my experiment, I've learned official names, in *The Diagnostic and Statistical Manual of Mental Disorders,* or *DSM,* which is the mental health bible: *hypoactive sexual desire disorder, female sexual arousal disorder, female orgasmic disorder, sexual aversion disorder, dyspareunia, vaginismus.* I have every hooha hang-up in the *DSM.*

Crucially, the *DSM* said hypnosis could help many of my challenges. It's my rationale for coming here. I cross my legs in my own miniskirt, black and longer than Dr. Fay's. My voice is almost robust:

"Okay, say the past *isn't* relevant? What about hypnosis to rewire me, you know, erotically? You said on the phone we could try hypnosis."

"I know," she sighs. "I know I did. But honestly? I don't think it'll help. I'd love it if it *did* help. But if you have no libido to begin with…"

"So I should just accept—this?" I am gesturing up and down my body.

"Yes!" says Dr. Fay. "Accept that you're *not* a sexual person. Stop putting so much pressure on yourself."

To argue with her assessment, I'd have to come up with a time before my dysfunctions began. All my wits can register is how my flaccid interest in lovemaking has ruined every relationship I've ever had. The last time Kurt and I argued about intimacy, he lay in our bed with tears rolling down his temples: "Why do you keep rejecting me?" I didn't have an answer for him. At the very least, I can get an answer. In my backpack is a journal. I had meant to take notes.

"So what do I do with my husband?" I ask, fishing for a pen I can't locate.

"Just have sex," Fay answers with a shrug.

"What do you mean?"

"Just. Have. Sex."

"When?"

"Whenever. Say your husband wants to get physical twice a week and you don't want to, you could *just have sex*. You don't have to like working out to go to the gym, do you?"

"I guess not."

"Of course you don't." Slowly, she leans forward till her forearms rest on her gold skirt. I can see a bit of cleavage. "I mean, you like being married, don't you?"

I blink. A lot. Not because what she's saying is shocking, but because I don't know why I'm pretending I'm shocked. It's how I always bedroom-existed until I got it into my skull I might mend myself. So what if her suggestion spits in the face of trauma recovery *and* consent *and* feminism? On the wall behind Dr. Fay's chair, I can see her license as someone whose expertise is wedlock.

"I love being married," I utter, with trembling again in my voice, in my bones.

"Good," says the dazzling female in front of me.

Dr. Fay's big light eyes make their way to a digital clock on her desk. "Well, we're just about out of time. Is there anything else?"

I gather my bag, my cardigan, the journal I took out but didn't write in. "No. That's it." I feel like she'd like me to pack up faster. "Thank you for seeing me." I rise from her blood red sofa.

"It was *my* pleasure," she says with glossy lips spread ear to ear. She believes she has solved my problem.

I suppose she has.

My curative project has been killed. The way I conceived of it, hypnosis—or at least faith—would plow a path for adventurous, multidimensional repair. I named this endeavor *The Pleasure Plan.*

On my feet, my mouth involuntarily mirrors hers, but *my* smile is fake. Then I remember something genuinely wonderful—Burger King. I noticed it in a shopping plaza down the road, right before I made a left into this office park. Suddenly, I can't wait to get out of there so I can order a chicken sandwich, crispy not grilled, with an order of fries—large, even though I'm a yoga teacher. I'll lick the grease off every finger until I'm sated and sleepy. Just the way I like it. I'll drive to my house half-asleep.

Taking a last glance around the office and at the hypnotist, who walks me into the (empty) waiting room, I say to myself: *She has got to be the worst therapist on the entire planet.* Consequently, I open the door to the hallway. It looks like a long tan tunnel. It is. A portal taking me back to my delicate life. I swing around.

"I want to try hypnosis," I announce. "I know you don't think it will help, but I want to do it anyway."

I have to start *somewhere.*

If I leave here without some implementation of my plan, I don't trust myself to seek out another hypnotist, or to advance. Perhaps my experiment has already stirred up desire—not for greasy things, but for its own freedom. And what I desire now is autosuggestion on a red leather couch with a therapist who may or may not be incompetent. I want her to change her mind about me.

"I'd like to schedule another appointment," I say, taking out my planner.

Reluctantly, she agrees.

Driving home to my husband, forgoing fast food, I try to imagine what lies beyond this day.

I can't see it, not yet, what it will take to ultimately, fully heal—fifteen kinds of practitioners, thirty pleasure-enhancing techniques. I never could have predicted the struggles Kurt and I would encounter. Or the aliveness that would permeate our lives.

I have no idea what's in store for me. All I know is that whatever happens, this visit has already altered my future—it has strengthened my body, my being, for hope.

Part 1
The Hump

1

How I Found the Love of My Life and Lost Him

To tell this story of sexual healing—to do it properly—we'll need to go back in time: five years before my meeting with the hypnotist.

On a sizzling July day in 2006, I stand inside the door of a French café in Washington, DC. I am meeting a stranger here.

My eyes scan the marble tables, cane-back chairs, and yellow walls adding cheerful contrast to the almost-black wood bar. The whole place smells like halibut and butter, and my own sharp sweat.

I spot my date. A balding, blond gentleman sits at a table near the window. He's older than his Match.com pictures, in which he appeared long and lean. He seems stockier. More solid. This is great for me. Once, when I was seven, a gusty wind lifted my feet in the air as I clung to a lamppost. Too often, I still feel I might blow away. It doesn't help that I'm tiny: 5'1" and petite.

I like him, I think, as I get closer to the man in the chair. Then I see the book in his hands. It's a play by a French-Caribbean playwright I studied in a college class, back in the eighties.

When Kurt sees me, he stands. An awkward handshake morphs into an awkward cheek kiss—both cheeks at his urging, French style. His skin feels soft. As he pulls away, I notice he's just a few inches taller, another plus. Tall men frighten me. I take in his orange T-shirt made of wicking fiber, his khakis. He appears stylish, but not hip. His profile said he was over fifty.

I like him, my head says again as I sit, but it isn't my head. It's a sensation at the top of my rib cage, like a lever that's been pulled in an upright position. For that scorching day (95 degrees, at least), I've chosen a cotton dress with pink and red roses. Its empire waist, directly below my breasts, presses in right where the internal, affirmative movement takes place. I don't know if it's muscle, organ, or nerves that create this visceral YES. But I trust it—even though it turns me into a monster.

I'm talking about the times this lever stayed down. It started when I was nineteen and committed myself to a lovely law student whose saliva had a weird consistency. Every weekend, we'd have sex on the single bed of his dorm room, each thrust another assault, before he'd lie on his back dozing. Ten minutes later (he was twenty-one), he'd want to do it all over again. Hating the rage these events inspired in me, wanting to cherish this nice person, I stayed for two years. And what about that guy who dominated my late thirties, the one whose skin had a vanilla-type odor I couldn't stand? Also, his face reminded me of a woman who lived on my block growing up. Sadly, she died of colon cancer. I dated this man for fifteen months because I despised my superficiality. In the two decades between these relationships, there were dozens quite similar—all with caring, funny, quirky men for whom I couldn't summon lust. I convinced myself I was a monstrous creature, in the reptilian family, with cold skin and blood.

Feeling nothing seemed a liability, but then I tried online dating. Landing in DC five years ago, I signed up on multiple platforms, where, I realized, scrolling past dudes was necessary. Rejection: a crucial part of the game. With practice, I learned early detection. These days, as I wait outside another Starbuck's (usually his choosing), my upper stomach can tell me the rendezvous will be disastrous from half a block away. Unfortunately, that's almost always my experience. But I no longer spend years with these fine fellows. I suppose I've just accepted my reptilian freeze.

That's why I've come out today, to this French restaurant, with an open mind but a forced smile at my ready, just in case.

Except . . . I don't have to pretend here. I'm grinning for real as Kurt tells me about the book he was perusing as I approached.

"Do you know Aimé Césaire?" he asks.

"I do. But I can't remember any of his plays. Is that a good one?"

"I just started it. But you're a playwright, right?"

"Yes." I nod my head and notice *his* head is very round and suddenly a little red. He has brought this drama to impress me.

Then he explains that when I walked up, he was purposely reading it upside down. It's a Kurt joke I don't yet understand. All I know is this: based on his effort, I'm pretty sure he also likes *me*.

Ten minutes later, my companion is savoring mussels in white wine while I graze on a veggie tartine. I'm having a glass of red wine too, though I rarely drink (I don't dig losses of control). Sipping as slowly as I can, I listen to Kurt talk about his work in the ethics office of an international organization. In our shared city of DC, lots of people have international development jobs. But I don't feel we're in Washington anymore. We've been transported to Paris. That was the reason we met here.

During an early exchange on the Match.com message app, Kurt wrote: "I picture us strolling through the Luxembourg Gardens. Afterward, we find ourselves on the street where Gertrude Stein lived. We stand across from her building, talking about literature. Then we take a long stroll to Île de la Cité, where there's an excellent ice cream shop..."

Taking in these lines, my breathing stopped. Just two months before, on a layover in Paris, I'd embarked on almost the exact same excursion. By myself.

Now, in this café, we are extending, as a team, our Francophile fantasy.

The French drink a lot of wine, don't they? I order another because I'm thousands of miles away from the young lawyer with funky saliva. I'm soaring above the handful of beaus who *did* grab my heart. There were three of them, and they all shared three traits: dark hair; a quick, mean wit; and an inability to love me. Maybe this blond man in the wicking orange shirt could also capture me—with his Caribbean drama, with his adorable bulbous nose.

I start speaking about my own plays. These are one-person pieces I perform myself. My most recent is about bad internet dating. "The title is *Stupid Frailty*," I tell him. "It's about a woman who's searching for a man she's physically attracted to, who's also attracted to her."

"Say more," responds my date, his chin between a thumb and index finger.

So I elaborate, extensively, as my hand gestures make larger and larger arcs until I become a windmill. Suddenly, one of my blades goes haywire, knocking my glass into the edge of the table. Dark red wine spills all over Kurt's light khakis.

Watching the stain spread like blood, I'm scared to gaze into this stranger's face. I'm waiting for him to respond with casual cruelty, like every other man I've risked liking.

Instead, Kurt laughs. "I'm so glad you did that. It's something I would have done!"

I notice his wispy hair, what's left of it, is sticking up erratically. I start rambling about living just up the hill. He asks if he can walk me home.

On the way, I feel the heat of his body next to mine on the sizzling street; it isn't too much. He takes my hand. When we get to my door, Kurt leans in to kiss me. It's a chaste peck on the lips, which seems appropriate—a perfect way to end the afternoon. But as he pulls away, I don't let him. It's not me doing this. It's my mouth, which plants back on his for another kiss. *This* smooch involves tongues and caresses of his back . . . his strong back.

And just like that, at forty-three, I'm having my first real relationship: I'm attracted and he's attracted back. Chemical reciprocity feels surreal. And this is gravy to our common interests—like French culture, theater, and speaking in fake accents. In those early weeks, we mash them together: "I zink zis relashohnsheep has poTENshahl!"

Even lovemaking is good in the initial months. Well, good by my standards. That means painful and no orgasm, but I want to do it anyway. It's one method of getting to know my paramour, who is mysteriously wonderful: *Look, he gives money to everyone on the street who asks for help. How did he find out about my niece's birthday without my telling him? How did his lips get so full and delicious?*

When I take Kurt to California to visit my brother, I corner Martin in his kitchen while Kurt's upstairs. My bro is standing there with his wife, his daughters, and other family. I grill everyone about this new person in my life: "What do you think of him?"

They all say the same thing, "We love him."

Me too, says the lever at the top of my ribs.

A year into our relationship, sex begins deteriorating. It's hard to pinpoint an exact date; physical intimacy has been extremely uncomfortable since my first consensual experiences, at seventeen. What I recall is a gradual awakening to change. But it's slight. *Is that more pain during intercourse? Yes, it's sharper, more like jabs. And burning. Was there always burning?*

It doesn't occur to me to discuss my vagina with friends, or a doctor. Yes, it's bad. It's also normal. This is my normal range.

Three years after our first date, Kurt proposes. It takes place during the curtain call of another of my one-person plays—in this piece I portray a man. As I'm bowing on the stage, I see my honey approach with a tremendous bouquet of flowers. Before I can absorb what's going on, he's right beside me, elevated above the crowd. He's down on one knee: "Will you marry me?"

"Is this part of the play?" audience members shout out.

I assure them it's not, taking off my man's wig. Then I turn back to Kurt's sweet, sweaty face. "Yes. YES," I tell my new fiancé as the crowd cheers.

Being Kurt's wife is exactly the right thing for me. What more is there?

I wish I could ask someone. Not *someone,* but my mom. In the lead-up to the wedding, I need so badly for Mom to reside on this earth again (she died fourteen years before) so I could ask her what's possible in a marriage.

"Don't go for passion." That's what she told me countless times growing up. These words usually came out right after I told her that I couldn't fall for saliva guy or another like him. She thought I was wrong to leave these men. "Don't go for passion," she'd repeat other times, glancing sideways at my dad, who'd once been tall, dark, and handsome until a neurological disease made him stooped, gray, and sallow. "It dies."

Having survived the Holocaust, my mother knew a lot about death. Which is to say she also knew a lot about life—that it was brutal at times, that it was saturated with evil, that it could be taken away at any moment. But also, it was damn fun to dance upon the earth, at least that's the way it *should* be for her children.

Despite two concentration camps (including Auschwitz), two Nazi ghettos, and a death march that began in Poland and ended hundreds of miles away in Germany, despite the murder of her parents and three siblings, my mother's favorite expression was "Get it!" Whenever I really wanted a treat—a doll with auburn hair growing out of a plastic knob on her skull, a rose-velvet jewelry box, a pair of silk chiffon shorts—she'd ask, "Do you love it?" If I responded, "Yes," her green eyes turned to emeralds. Then she'd make two fists under her chin, like a little girl watching cookies bake. Even with her hands closed, I could see they were chafed by peroxide she used on people's hair, by bleach she scrubbed into old men's toilets—her odd jobs. "Get it," she'd announce with a wisdom gained in Holocaust hell. My own personal Viktor Frankl.

When we tried giving *her* gifts, my mother threw them out, saying, "I don't need nothing." Yet, mixed with her preferred deprivation, I think she'd once known lust with my dad. I wasn't sure.

So many times before the wedding I imagine sitting in Mom's messy kitchen, drinking coffee boiled on the stove, Euro-style. She's wearing a big hat, even in the house, and one false eyelash is falling off. Show tunes are playing in the background. I ask: *Even if passionate ecstasy does fade and die, shouldn't great sex be there in the beginning? Isn't there more that I can scoop out of life and suck on with abandon?*

In lieu of this conversation, I feel lost. My married friends certainly offer advice—the road to wedded bliss. But their tips are tinged with bitterness, their own disappointment. I buy bridal magazines to find untainted guidance. I pile them on my bed.

Kurt and I get married in a civil ceremony that's beautiful, absolutely perfect. We opt out of a lavish wedding, choosing, alternatively, a romantic getaway in Europe, six months down the pike. A honeymoon in Rome.

Then, before we know it, we're here.

We're in Rome, after a long flight, and we are naked—my idea.

Because my lover's lips are full. They're on my shoulder now, the right one. I want him to kiss the left one too, but he doesn't. He chooses the right ear lobe instead, tongue swirling.

"Wait a second." I jump up.

"Where are you going?"

"Just wait."

Cold air clings to skin as I dash into the bathroom of our antique-filled hotel room. On a small mahogany table, next to a bidet I can't wait to use, next to the pedestal sink, is exactly what I'm after—a scrunchie. The red velvet kind nobody wears anymore. Butterfly clips be damned! Scrunchies are the best way to turn my brown curly hair into a ball, making room for tiny nibbles. Oh yeah, I'm also dodging.

But I'm back now. Reclining on the quilted gold comforter, splayed on top, I'm nude, like before, but more so somehow. Kurt's artfully shaped lips land on mine. But now they're too loose, or too big, taking up my mouth and some chin. Also, a bit of nostril.

To escape, I place my ear on his swimmer's chest, where I listen to his heart. It's fast, tapping out rapture, hunger. My own beats sound irregular, and not just because of a murmur. Suddenly, tears form in my chest, a wave of sadness that I hope will crest and fall before it makes its way to my eyes. It's stupid to crave more, even if it *is* your honeymoon. I swallow hard to scare away the sadness, which travels into my throat anyway. It squeezes, achingly *Where's my rapture-hunger?*

I jump up again.

"You keep going away," my groom pouts, holding out muscular arms that like to fix things.

"I'll just be a minute."

The room is dark (it must be midnight), but a yellow shaft of light seeps in from a piazza below. This glow is amplified by all the gold in this suite—carpet, satiny comforter, curlicue handles on the Pledge-shine dresser. I see what I'm after. I see my suitcase, still unpacked.

On the floor, kneeling, my hands slip inside, searching among my summer dresses and skirts, until I find it. A modest bundle wrapped tightly in fresh, pink tissue paper. Its contents: one baby doll nightgown (black gauze); two Cosabella thongs (black mesh); and a tube of rose-water body cream that comes in its own gold foil box. My trousseau.

Refusing the bridal shower my friends wanted to throw me because it was too much fuss, I treated myself to a high-end department store, spending money I didn't have. *I'm a bride, finally, at forty-six!*

Then I assembled my own version of what brides take on their wedding night—featured in so many mags. In the olden days, it was white linen sheets and slightly sheer nightgowns. It was tablecloths and crinolines. Everything was starched and smelled of violet water a great-aunt had sprayed before placing these items, lovingly, in a cedar chest.

"Just one more sec," I yell to Kurt, taking my modern, tissue-paper trousseau into the bathroom, where I slip into the baby doll negligee. The bottom ruffle tickles my upper thighs but this garment makes me feel calmer, like I'm wearing a burka. Albeit, mine is short and sheer.

"Where'd you get *that*?" my honey asks when I return to his toasty sheets. Immediately, he peels off the straps of my nightie, kissing down to the nipples.

Nerves pop just beneath the skin; too many of them, setting off a reflex in my stomach that wants to rebel, or expel something, possibly vomit. He starts going down on me. The nerve frenzy from this activity is worse. Like four thousand bees on my spinal cord, buzzing all at once. It's always been like this. *Who doesn't love cunnilingus?* Yet another reason I'm defective. I pull my lover back up.

"What's wrong?" he asks.

"Nothing."

Then I rush into intercourse, even though I'm not ready. I'm never ready. I dry up completely, which feels like a fingernail scraping off tissues, layer by layer. We've tried lube, which hasn't helped very much. Is this an age thing? I've heard about inner skin shriveling up after a certain age, but how could this apply to me? I've never been juicy.

Kurt is on top of me, pumping away.

One. Two. Three. *Ow.*

Four. *Ow.*

Five. *Ow.*

Six. *Ow. Fuck.* Not good fuck.

After a few more thrusts, my groom climaxes and rolls on his back. It takes a moment for his eyes to open.

"How was it?" he asks with uncertainty in his voice.

Searching for words, I give up right away. There's never been language attached to these experiences—not with Kurt, not with any human for the past thirty years.

"Good," I say, lying, but almost believing it myself.

The next morning, I bolt awake realizing I've got a problem, an extensive one—my bras do not match my panties. I'm talking about everything I own, including my trousseau, especially my trousseau. *I mean, a baby doll nightgown. How juvenile. No wonder I'm not transported to erotic realms.* I need to go shopping. Today. All day. Now.

Unfortunately, we have other plans. A trip to historic sites, which are, you know, a big deal. Mostly, these are elaborate churches Kurt will be introducing me to. Rome was my husband's chrysalis. In the eighties, he lived here for a year, transitioning from Midwest autoworker's son into garlic-frying intellectual. Every crevice of this town played a part in his evolution. He's eager to share his favorite corners with me, to show me who he is. And I want to see him. But I also want him to see me, to see myself—in a synchronized bra and underwear set!

While Kurt's in the shower singing "'O Sole Mio" for my benefit, I linger in the golden bed, clenching and unclenching my toes. I need to suppress my stupid urge to shop. Hasn't retail therapy always failed? What about those eighteen pairs of shoes I bought when my mom died, purchased in six weeks? I tried six colonics to offset this expenditure, but the math didn't work. Everything was put on a Visa I never paid off. Didn't I ruin my credit for years? Of course I did. It's time to just be present with my husband.

An hour later, we're in a Renaissance-perfect piazza behind our hotel so my fella can photograph the Fountain of the Four Rivers, a sprouting sculpture so white and intricate it looks like it was made of plaster. Four enormous, carved river gods comprise the bulk of it, each mounting a curvy stone wave. In the middle of this action, an obelisk rises, like an arrogant phallus, ninety or one hundred feet into the sky.

It makes my ears pulse with mad, hot blood.

As Kurt points out the landmark's attributes, I focus on *his* attributes and breathe. I marvel at his cute blond hair and blue eyes; the way that, despite his fair complexion, he can totally tan. He's like a short member of the Beach Boys. Standing there in a blue button-down shirt, beige shorts, white sneakers, and black photography bag slung across his toned upper body, he reminds me of a dad not addicted to Budweiser or porn.

"Ready for church?" my wholesome honey asks, stowing away his camera.

"You bet," I declare loudly, pushing away the silky undergarments dancing around in my head. Something else gets booted out too: an intruder. It's no use. He's all over this plaza, at least his image is, in the souvenir shops lining this square—the pope. *I won't let him destroy my honeymoon.*

It's just an unfortunate coincidence.

On top of everything else, by some weird happenstance, the current pope, Benedict the XVI, looks exactly—I mean exactly—like one of the men who molested me when I was four. The resemblance is shocking. Same white hair. Same sunken eyes. Same stubby hands that used to undress me.

Kurt knows all about my abuse. I told him shortly after we met. I've told everyone I know. I've been talking about this shit, openly, for decades. But there are aspects of this complexity I still cannot articulate.

The first time I ever said out loud I'd been molested, I was sitting in front of my house, on the curb. It was on a hot August day, the summer I turned six, two years after the abuse began. My brother Martin and I were sorting rocks we had found in the street.

"This one's for Grandpa," I said, holding up a smooth gray stone with a pointy top. It looked like something that belonged in a cemetery. I said this because my grandfather had recently died. This was my way of processing grief. I assumed my only sibling—who was two years older and knew *everything*—would understand what I was trying to say. Instead, Martin's face puffed up.

"Take that back," he responded. "What you said was bad."

I had disrespected the memory of our grandfather. *But how? What did I say?* It didn't matter. My brother's condemnation sent explosions throughout my body, blasts that were hollowing me out. I had to do something—to save myself, or hurt him, which seemed like the same thing. So I told him about our neighbor—a completely different grandpa—the grandfather of our friend, Tammy. "You know what Tammy's grandfather did?" I went on to elaborate.

In my six-year-old mind, telling him this horrible news was retribution. I knew he wouldn't be able to handle it. I was right. Martin's skull blew up until it became grotesque: a huge, raging balloon. He started yelling, "You'd better tell Mommy. Now!"

My first response was to scan our dead-end block full of trees, seeking a path of escape. Largely unsupervised, I knew excellent backyard hiding places. But I was trapped. My big brother had given me an order. An obedient child, I did what older folks commanded.

Stepping inside my house, I cursed myself. *I don't want to tell anyone. That's why I didn't tell anyone. Why did I tell him? Something bad is going to happen.*

Shadows of violence scurried across my mind. Mom was always insinuating danger could erupt in our home because Dad was "mentally ill." A few times, my mother called the cops, screaming to the police that my father had threatened her with a knife. I never saw a sharp object during these encounters, so I didn't know whom to believe as we all stood around. Should I side with my mom's vibrating body or my dad's embarrassed laugh?

What if there is a knife? I thought as I searched for my mother in the basement, backyard, and living room before locating her. Mom was making the bed in her miniscule room off the kitchen. Dad slept in another part of the house; I was too young to analyze this arrangement. I ordinarily loved this room because of the textured wallpaper—red and blue velvet stripes ran down a white background—but that day the stripes popped out like the varicose veins on Mom's legs. She said she'd gotten these when she gave birth to me. My mother seemed so rushed as she tucked in the corners of the fitted sheet, which was also the color of veins.

"Martin told me to tell you something," I said.

"Tell me what?" she asked, not glancing up from her task.

I wanted to answer but had run out of words—forever? I watched the flat sheet she was fluffing over the bed. Each time she brought it down, the puff of air felt good because she was sweating. Maybe it would make her stop sweating.

The breeze also brought a whiff of laundry detergent, which

somewhat masked onions from our kitchen. Our house smelled like old people, so said my friends. This made sense since strangers often thought my mother was my grandmother. It was the housedresses and Polish-Yiddish accent I'd never heard on another mother. It was the onions, in the kitchen and often on Mom's breath. Just then, paralyzed in the doorway, I wasn't close enough to her to find out if this was currently the case.

"You have something to tell me, or you don't have something to tell me?" she asked.

Whatever I said was brief. Just a sentence, I think.

Mom sighed hard. Then she fixed her green eyes on me. People said I had a matching set. I'd never seen hers look so ugly. There was too much scrunching around them and they were watery like she was tearing up. But it couldn't be true; my mother never cried. In fact, the voice that came out of her was angry: "That's what men are like! Don't go *near* him."

As an obedient child, I listened. For years, I constructed schemes and elaborate systems, to get away from Tammy's grandfather.

I'm still running away from this man. But differently. That's what I can't put into words. How, over the years, this abuser became part of my body, my vagina, wreaking havoc there. I got used to him though—his benign creepiness. I learned I could tolerate his damage as long as I pretended he wasn't there. That's how things stood until 2005, the year Benedict became pope, five years before my honeymoon.

Overnight, I was inundated by his shocking, huge head. It seemed like my tormenter—in holy form—had risen from the dead. I turned off television sets, closed internet windows, and clicked out of news-paper articles, with some exceptions. I relished the many stories impli-cating him, or just investigating his role, in the growing sex abuse scandal roiling the Catholic Church. I shared this rage with no one, preferring to screech in my mental belfry: *How many children have been molested? How many, Benedict?*

Did I know that my rage was displaced? Sure. But I loved having this target.

I still love it.

Or I did, before I got to Rome. Before I got to this plaza, where I am not getting off on being triggered—because I'm trying to get off the other way! Is that too much to ask?

The thing is, this man-god is EVERYWHERE. As Kurt and I con-tinue our journey to the first church he's trying to show me, we are confronted with more souvenir shops every fifty feet. Posters. Key chains. Postcards. Ashtrays.

I grab Kurt's hand because I will not succumb to this assault. There's so much else to focus on. Cobblestones must be navigated in my red wedge sandals. We're trekking between, around, so many fresh-morning tourists yelling in Spanish, in Japanese, in Polish. *Is that Czech or Polish?* Next, my husband is talking about the church itself. It houses black-veined marble obtained from Africa. This sounds intriguing until Kurt relays that a long-ago pope laid claim to this precious material—because he could.

Another fucking pope.

Without warning, my imagination cuts to a priest in a shower. A shivering boy is there, a recent feature in the news. Other media pred-ators begin rotating in my head—trusted coaches, beloved teachers, someone's bullying cousin—a dizzying display. I halt, noticing my eyes have closed and I'm drenched.

"Are you okay?" Kurt asks.

"Give me a minute" I say, pulling in air with suddenly half-working lungs. A shaking hand clears sweat away from under my eyes, and down my arms. "I feel nauseous," I tell Kurt, but I'm not sure why. It's not true. Though now that I've mentioned it, my belly goes a little wobbly.

Kurt stands with me, stroking my shoulder.

"I think it's the heat," I offer as explanation because why ruin his day with this displaced, blasphemous rage? Kurt knows explicit details of my molestation. But that was forty years in the past! And not by priests, or the holiest man on earth. My husband left the church, but his family is still devoutly Catholic.

"Do you want to sit down?" he asks.

When I decline, he leaves to buy me a bottle of water. I'm relieved to be alone, even though the soot-stained building I'm leaning against is the only thing keeping me upright, even though my pink, flowered skirt sticks to my butt, and my red tank top, betraying its yoga studio logo, maliciously chafes my back.

After Kurt returns, I gulp his offering, the cooling liquid, with my lids open to force out smirking perverts, who have merged into a single man—the pope. I've got the wrong guy.

The destination church is right in front of us, my husband explains, tucked inside a plaza that's partly in view. He thinks if I can make it inside the edifice and sit down, I'll feel better. I open my eyes to see what he means. And that's when I notice it—pure magic, like an apparition. "What's that?" I ask.

Almost where we're standing, directly across the street, is a shiny shop with a glass and chrome façade. Together, Kurt and I sound out the name: "In-ti-miss-i-mi."

"What does it mean?" I ask as if I'm blind to all the sensual lingerie in the window.

"Intimacy, I think."

"Do you mind if I go in?" The question itself invigorates me.

"Now?" Kurt asks with spiked brows. "I thought you didn't feel good."

"I'm better now."

He frowns. I know how it must look. We've been traveling to someplace sacred, not a depot of pricey merchandise made by Chinese laborers choking to death on factory toxins.

"I'll just be a minute," I say, throwing the oppressed workers under a bus.

"You won't be a minute," he counters, knowing my filthy plastic habits. "Why don't we go to church and swing back here after?"

"No. Let's split up. You go there," I say, indicating the plaza that contains the religious building. "And I'll go shopping." As soon as it comes out of my mouth, it sounds sacrilegious, shallow.

Kurt considers the equation nonetheless—not so much with his skull but with his jaw, which grinds when he's tense.

"Fine." He sighs and checks his elaborate sports watch. "Thirty minutes?"

"Thirty minutes," I say, bobbing my head up and down like I'm a doll on the dashboard of his car.

The second he leaves, I enter Intimissimi. The space is blindingly, stunningly white. The track lighting, the floors, the walls, and display tables are the same shade, a tasteful concoction. A tasty one too. It's like standing inside a dollop of whipped cream.

I don't say it to myself. I don't have to: *I feel safe*. I stroke silk camisoles and silky T-shirts hanging on a rack near the door. What I really want to fondle is the atmosphere itself. It smells like honeysuckle and lemon and white things mixed together with pink. I could stay here all day, but what kind of person chooses underwear over famous artistic treasures that have nothing to do with abuse from a million years ago?

A person like me.

When I was younger, in my twenties, I collected garter belts and stockings. I'd put them on under skirts that had some swing. Then I'd walk down the streets of New York City feeling insouciant. (I remember loving that word back then: *insouciant.*) My free spirit, my prance, the sway of my hips were fabulous until some schmuck gaped at me or made a comment. I didn't want sex. I wanted to be sexy.

All these years later, I'm still confused—these tracks run parallel but don't necessarily touch.

Aren't they supposed to touch?

I try connecting to my simple goal this morning: buy some freakin' lingerie. I wander around, studying posters lining the vanilla walls. They show me young women with uncovered midriffs, pushed-up orbs, and limbs going on for miles (I mean, kilometers). Within reach is a jellybean assortment of thongs on a huge, round table; I finger each one. I stare at balconettes—brassieres I've never heard of, in spite of my undergarment research. The name evokes a veranda where people in crisp linen sip Chianti under the stars. If my boobs were adorned with Italian sophistication, would I be delivered to that veranda?

Suddenly, I spot Kurt.

He's on the other side of the glass windows playing with his phone, sort of. Though the iPhone came out three years before, he's sticking with his flip. He won't buy a new item unless the old one is broken. I wonder if he'll replace *me* when he discovers the extent to which I am broken.

When he sees me, he lifts up his wrist so I can see his watch. I leave my paradise empty-handed, unmoored.

Strolling home from our day of religious relics, we pass musicians playing violins on the embankment of the Tiber River, which runs through this entire city—the most romantic in the world. I suggest that my groom spend a day without me.

"Freedom isn't such a bad thing," I say. "The things that you like are not the things that I like."

"What does *that* mean?" My husband stops abruptly. His eyes, magnified through his not-so-hip wire-rimmed glasses, are immense, bloodshot.

"It doesn't mean anything," I say, wishing I could take back my suggestion, the implication we should spend our honeymoon apart. "Forget I mentioned it."

"No, it means something," he insists. "If you don't like the way we're spending our vacation, just say it instead of being passive-aggressive."

"I'm not passive-aggressive," I say in a high-pitched voice.

"Yes, you are. You don't speak up, and then you make that face."

"What face?"

"That disgusted face."

"I love our vacation," I assure Kurt, as I take his arm and usher us back to our hotel bed.

The next thing I do is max out three credit cards. It doesn't transpire all at once though. And to be fair, I already had high balances on each of these plastic rectangles, due to my retail therapy. I've had enough *actual* therapy to know my spending is compensating for loss. Also, it's how I've supplemented my paltry income teaching theater and yoga. Whatever the rationale, I'm always shocked when the bill comes.

I'm not thinking of debt, however, when I first return to the creamy paradise. In the fitting room, studying myself in a massive gilded mirror, I try on a royal blue balconette. *A balconette.* The matching panty is scratchy, but it makes my stomach appear flat because of its high waist. Both pieces have an overlay of white lace, like curtains on a Victorian home, or dense mosquito netting.

Running my hand from sternum to pubic bone, I begin conjuring what I most want from Italy. A reddening of my pale cheeks. A hardening of the nipples. I see them poking, ever so slightly, through the armored lace of the bra. Maybe I was right to search for matching. Perhaps symmetry *can* heal me. A phrase from one of my Eastern philosophy books pops into my mind: *As above, so below.*

When Kurt meets me back at the hotel, even before he puts down his knapsack, I parade around the room in my outfit, running my fingers sensually over my breasts ... my thighs ... my ankles. With each caress, I'm transformed into a poster vixen in a lingerie shop. I'm finally sexy.

A similar scene plays out all week, but the ending never changes—no matter which new get-up adorns me. Inevitably, that costume comes off and a man is on top of me. The vamp on tiptoes is replaced by a person whose vagina is ugly and aching. In these moments, I'm all alone with a private phrase: *Get off me. Get off me.*

Do I like or love Kurt in these moments?

I don't know. I'm too far away to notice.

Tips for *Your* Pleasure Plan

Something to Try:

Journal for five to ten minutes, setting a timer. During that time, construct a perfect romantic vision for yourself. It can be meeting the partner of your dreams, making love in a way that really feeds your soul, or anything that turns you on. Don't be afraid of being too racy, sweet, tender, animalistic, or any combination! When the timer goes off, add this sentence to what you wrote: "I deserve this."

Journal Prompts:

1. Do you feel "broken?" If so, what do you mean by this word or any phrase associated with it?

   _____

   _____

   _____

2. What bedroom challenges do you face?

   _____

   _____

   _____

3. Do you have an intuition about what might help?

   _____

   _____

   _____

Oprah Wants Me to Get a Dildo

I think the answer is sex toys.

As soon as Kurt and I return to the States, I'm excited to buy some help of this nature. It's stupid, I know, trying to purchase my way out of these struggles—again—but I don't know how else to activate my desire. Or arousal. *Do I know anything at all about desire and arousal?*

Also, I'm terrified of toys. Isn't that reason enough to investigate?

On the web, there's no shortage of these items. But I find most shapes and functions stupefying. I'm thinking of dismissing this option. But while walking home from teaching during that same week, I randomly wander into a used bookstore on my path. Right away I see it, near the door, on a peeling rack. It's a coffee-table-sized book with a handsome couple embracing on the cover, called *Loving Sex*. Making sure no one is close by, I pick up the guide, and sure enough, I see glossy photos of couples engaged in all kinds of erotic play, including the use of sex toys. There's even explanatory text!

Suddenly, it feels like neighbors are everywhere; this is a neighbor-hood shop. I put the book exactly where I found it but stay close by, my curiosity and nervous system ignited. Only then do I notice the author, Dr. Laura Berman, a famous sex therapist frequently featured on Oprah's show and in her magazine. Ms. Winfrey, as most people know, was sexually abused. From these fragments I conclude: Oprah is dying for me to get a vibrator.

Or a dildo.

Or a vibrating dildo.

Or, at least a book that helps me understand this technology.

But getting in Oprah's way are all the fucks I give about the people around me.

Getting in her way is the guy behind the register.

I barely noticed him when I first entered, but now that I'm think-ing of acquiring this mating manual, he has my full attention. He's a middle-aged hipster stuck in the eighties with dyed-black hair; a red, plaid shirt; and a spiky leather cuff. He's like dudes I went to high school with—*in the actual eighties*. These boys radiated hot confidence about obscure, fantastic music. In their presence, I felt like a child *sans* boobs or my first pubic hair.

I pace the long aisles of this cavernous store. Harsh fluorescents follow me like a spotlight. I imagine everyone can see my sluttiness and lack of sluttiness, simultaneously. I want to rip off my red car-digan, throwing it on the dirty green carpet. I want to stomp on this outer layer, as a gesture. A gesture of what? Maturity? The right to be erotic? Returning to *Loving Sex*, setting it into my moist hands, I clutch it all the way to the cashier.

"Oh, you're buying it?" Hipster challenges in low tones the instant I place my book on his register. His deep voice has a no-problem-man tone like he smokes a lot of pot. "I didn't get a chance to even look at it."

In the five years I've been coming to this shop, these are the most words—cumulatively—any employee has ever said to me.

"Sorry," I spit out. "But you know it's Oprah's . . . I mean the author . . . she's a sex therapist . . . Oprah's. It's really comprehensive."

To prove my point, I start leafing through the book, which suddenly smells like it was buried under torn clothes in a damp basement. That scent might be coming from the shopkeeper. He has joined me in turning pages, with fingers yellow from weed or fungus. *Why is he touching my book?* My intestines quiver as we browse through couples biting, tickling, and licking each other. After we get to the last page, he conducts our financial transaction. His relaxed hand is that of someone lighting a post-coital cigarette.

Handing back my credit card, he says: "Do you want a bag? Or will you just . . ." He's holding *Loving Sex* in front of his chest, like a big letter A.

"I'm not ashamed," I say, peering directly into his black eyes for the first time. I hold his gaze and breathe. I sprout breasts.

I also take a plastic bag.

At home, Kurt, noticing my sack, asks me what I purchased. It's a casual remark; he's just making chit-chat. Yet when I show him, his eyebrows go up and down like those of Groucho Marx.

I'm fatigued by my own courage, or that nail fungus. So I decide to just get it over with. "How about a quickie?" I suggest. There's not enough time for me to summon the wee dose of turn-on I can sometimes muster. There's never enough time. I'm as dry as an old corpse.

That's why after my husband leaves for work the next morning, I push aside the fourth-grade drama lesson on my desk that's due by the end of the day (K–12 teaching is another of my jobs). Time for a mini break. Letting myself swivel in my office chair, pressing my groin (my loins?) into the cherry red cushion, I go straight to the center of Laura Berman's book, where the toy action starts. As I mentioned, this large, beautifully photographed guide has wisdom regarding all manner of sensuality. But right now, I'm sticking with the gadgets.

On page 185, a hot-pink rod pokes out from a black gal's panties. Dr. Berman tells me, like a well-informed sister, that this is a dildo without vibration, a tool for pure penetration. My elbows press into my ribs, more tense contraction than self hug. I do like the color, though. It coordinates nicely with the rose walls adorning this entire apartment, a color that doesn't let on that a man lives here. I keep telling Kurt we should paint our home, make it more masculine, and he agrees. Then I postpone. I think it's because I'm still learning to be feminine.

Loving Sex is helping. On another page, a blond gal in a green bra (exclusively) reclines on a bed. She's holding a silver-toned vibrator resembling a tube of lipstick. I love lipstick. Will I love the clitoral stimulation Berman promises with this device? I'm not sure. Most clitoral sensations are overwhelming, though I can't fathom why. I have to train my lady parts, no doubt. Shall it be the rosy dick, the buzzing lipstick, a glass dildo, a ridged phallus, and other inventions I find here?

I'll get them all.

Suddenly, an elevator drops in my stomach. It's the credit card bills sitting in the top drawer of this cheap IKEA desk. They itemize the lingerie I bought in Rome, thousands of dollars of genital-inspired debt. Monthly payments are already a struggle.

No more debt, I swear it to myself, along with this pledge: *I'll scrape up money for one appliance to use privately while my spouse is at the office.* I just know its magic will bring me back from the dead.

I just have to choose. As I go back to the photos, running my hands over each one, nothing interests me. If I'm honest, truly honest, every damn object elicits the same response: a full-body wince. In other words, maybe the answer is *not* sex toys.

Could it merely be a matter of getting turned on?

If so, there are hundreds of other tasteful, simulated sex images in this book. A gray-haired paunchy guy enters his paunchy female partner from the rear; two long, tall, model-types (he brunette, she platinum) go at it on a desk; a lesbian couple kisses. I scrutinize this titillation, hunting for my own flutter or tingle or buzz. A hum?

Nothing.

Why aren't I aroused? I keep asking myself this question until an angry mob takes over my head. It wants to know: *Who are these people?*

I'm turning two, three pages at a time, but I'm searching for something entirely different now. I'm searching for . . . me. Aren't there individuals who have hurdles like I do? Where are we? Why can't we exist alongside that paunchy (and non-paunchy) rear entry? Don't we get to wear a sequined mask?

It's not like Berman's book avoids struggles. She's got a robust section on STIs, on low libido, on age-related sex decline. But I'm still not seeing myself. Not the full scope of my issues. Time to close her gorgeous book and open the unkempt internet, where I do find mention of dysfunction—*sexual dysfunction*—a phrase I've never used in my life. However, most paragraphs focus on erectile troubles.

Erections. Erections. Erections.

Dangerously neglecting my drama lesson, I keep following links. These lead to other links. Eventually, I wind up on a cyber road that delivers me somewhere strange.

Vaginismus.

It's a lady problem that makes me burst out laughing. *What dumb fuck would burden a woman with such a horribly-named disorder?* But then I read the symptoms: pain and burning with intercourse, difficult or impossible penetration, an inability to use tampons. "Vaginismus is a condition marked by involuntary contractions of the vaginal muscles, largely the pubococcygeus, or PC muscle. It is brought on by fear of penetration."

Every cell in my being stands at attention—little cell hands on little cell hearts—making a declaration: *This is what's wrong with me. This is what I have!*

By now, I've magnetically merged with a website devoted to vaginismus. I'm staring into the faces of frowning, handsome couples and their smiling (also handsome) counterparts. The latter have, presumably, used the remedy they sell on this site—hard, plastic dildos they call dilators. These white cylinders, hollow inside and made of the same material as a cheap radio, come in graduated sizes. The smallest has the dimensions of a finger, while the largest is the width and length of an "average" erect penis.

The screen blurs as fat tears cover my eyes. By the time they run down my cheeks, I am realizing—for the first time—what happened back in college with Jeremy, an early boyfriend.

Jeremy was the friend of Alex, the one I really had a crush on. He even asked me on a date. Born in Greece, Alex had a broad jaw, a permanent tan, and triangular eyebrows that resembled structures on the façade of the Parthenon. It was raining the day he explained, on the stairs of a Neo-Greek building, he was going back to his ex-girlfriend. This was before we actually went out.

She had cheated but was sorry. Yada yada. I suspected the real culprit was my breath. In addition to having a fake tooth jutting out from a bite plate—the result of being hit by a car when I was ten—I'd recently been told by a new dentist that I had halitosis due to gum disease. Evidently, my prior dentist hadn't just been a sadist; he'd been a moron. At seventeen, I'd never had my teeth cleaned. So when Alex described his situation, I said I understood because I did. *Why would anyone want to be with me?*

And yet, my Greek god had a friend; he even arranged things. Jeremy did not make my insides vibrate, not at all. But romance with someone I desired seemed impossible. Didn't Alex just prove that? Jeremy was good enough. Then, after a few weeks of courtship, he grew on me. I became enamored with his ginormous, wavy-brown hair; his neatly trimmed fingernails; and the creased jeans he ironed himself. He enticed me to fall in love with him.

Since we went to a commuter college, and lived at home with our respective parents, our intimate experiments took place in his parents' basement. I was terrified of everything, but Jeremy was patient. Using the same meticulousness that made sure his pants were perfectly pressed, he taught me fellatio. This oral action didn't freak me out as much as I thought it would. However, when his fingers were inside me, I became convinced open wounds were lining my inner walls. I never told Jeremy to stop because I figured since I'd been abused, there were consequences. Permanent consequences.

Yet, despite disliking poking, I had no reason to believe making love wouldn't be ecstatic, like in the movies. One day Jeremy announced his parents were going away for the weekend. I was wet for a week waiting for it to happen. Finally, amidst paneling and mildew, both of which went back decades, I lay on a faded plaid couch, while Jeremy put on *Deja Vu*, an album by Crosby Stills Nash and Young. These were the days before CDs, so Jeremy had to keep jumping up to flip sides. That was the least of our worries. We couldn't do it. It just wouldn't go in. With condoms, without—it didn't matter.

For weeks, we tried to get it in. To get it. In. To get. It. In. There was no budging. Jeremy, who had little bedroom experience himself, pleaded with me to see a gynecologist. I explained I didn't know any because of my family's bizarre relationship with the medical community. Blame it on Mengele. Josef Mengele, the "Angel of Death," presided over medical aspects of Auschwitz, where my mother was a prisoner in 1944. My mom said he would whistle a tune while waiting for cattle cars to pull up. Then he'd separate those able to work from the rest, whom he sent to the ovens. We didn't know what happened to Mom's mother, two of her sisters, and a brother. It's very possible Mengele sent them to the ovens. We shunned doctors in my home. I'm lucky Mom took me to that dimwit dentist.

Jeremy continued pressing though. Scanning the yellow pages at the school library (as one did back then), I found an OB/Gyn near our college, a Brazilian woman with a messy blond bob. Her hazel eyes were oversized and kind as I spelled out my difficulty. This was pre-exam, still dressed, seated on her steel table. What came next was…unprecedented. The speculum felt medieval, the way it cranked me wider and wider. I was terrified she'd rip me apart.

"Relax," said the Brazilian in a breezy tone, like we were lounging on the beach in Rio.

Her directive involved my knees, which kept snapping shut. I'm not sure how I managed to let her take a peek, but she did.

"Everything's normal," she informed me with a little laugh. Then, still caught up in merriment, she added. "Next time you're with your boyfriend, have some wine. And relax."

"Okay," I said quickly so she would remove the metal monster. Back in my skirt and undies, I only listened as she got more specific with her remedy: "Have some wine. Some *red* wine." On a prescription pad, she wrote down an item important to pair with the vintage—K-Y Jelly.

I had no idea what this was, but my drugstore did. When I gave my doctor's scribble to the girl behind the counter, she screeched in a Brooklyn voice loud enough for the whole line of people to hear: "K-Y Jelly? You don't need a prescription for K-Y Jelly!"

Most of the other customers were old men, grandfathers. It took hours until my blazing face returned to baseline. Ultimately, I was glad to have this assistance. It complemented beer and Burgundy, vodka and Long Island Ice Teas. I took the doctor's advice to heart: if I wanted to screw, I needed to be blotto. Two months after my appointment, *eight months* after our initial attempt, Jeremy and I consummated our relationship. It was excruciating, that night and each time we tried for weeks afterward.

Then, the discomfort subsided.

Though not completely.

Never completely.

Three decades later, gaping at the vaginismus website, still planted at my desk, I realize my condition has never gotten better, not substantially. I find out that what I have is actually known as primary vaginismus. This is when tight pelvic floor muscles have never known another state. Secondary vaginismus means a person has had normal PC function, but then these muscles seize up after a genital shock (like surgery).

Sure, I've learned to dismantle the barrier, partially, allowing penetration. But entry hurts, nonetheless. And once deep thrusting starts, my sanctum freaks out in a completely different way. It's like being a virgin every single time. Sorry, Madonna, this is not sexy.

My vagina is busted. I should be happy I understand why. Rather, I pace my apartment as accusations bounce around my skull: *Why have I never heard of this infirmity? You're telling me not a single person who treated me—shrink or gynecologist—had knowledge about this?*

It's as if, for three decades, I had a dislocated shoulder but not a single soul knew what to call it—so they couldn't fix it. Then one day, a person *who actually knew about joint injuries* examined my arm and said, "No worries, Missy, your shoulder is dislocated. I'll just pop the ball back in its socket."

If it *had* been my shoulder, would I have decided that challenges with one part of the body made me a defective human being? Probably not. Yet, that's what I've done my whole life.

All of a sudden, I'm dying to talk to Kurt about this. I have to tell him everything—because it isn't him. It isn't even me. It's a medical thing. And it's curable.

I'm not sure how I'll justify my lying. I need to climb toward truth nonetheless—now that I have truth. Vaginismus. *That fucking name . . .* I start laughing again, this time with my head thrown back like a madwoman, but it's no longer the nomenclature I'm thinking of. My most profound sadness and shame, the trauma haunting me since I was victimized as a toddler, are you telling me it all amounts to a spazzy set of muscles?

Whatever it is, at least I've found a remedy—those therapeutic dildos. Kurt and I could snuggle on the mattress while I insert the littlest one. Then the brokenness that has been mine for so long will be his too.

See? I was right. Sex toys.

I don't tell Kurt, though, not right away. First, I grill my friends at a trendy Italian eatery that has too much chilly chrome and freezing white vinyl.

"Vagi-what?" exclaims my friend Gayle.

"Vaginismus," I whisper, making sure random people in this echoing, cold restaurant can't hear us. Gayle and I and our buddy Stacey are huddled at a corner table. Gayle, her blond hair perfectly highlighted and blown out, has come prepared in her stylish cashmere cape. This born leader, who heads up a women's health organization, knows female things. She's the real reason I postponed the hubby confession, so I could acquire her insight.

Disturbingly, she's never heard of my condition. Maybe she didn't hear it right. "Vag-i-NIS-mus," I repeat.

"Vagina Christmas?" asks Stacey. In her Indian skirt and oversized sweater, she's the earth mama of our group.

I assure them both that whatever a Vagina Christmas is—and it does sound festive, even to a curly haired Jewish girl like me—this is its evil twin.

I don't ask my friends what's itching in my skull. Do they also have discomfort sometimes? I don't bring this up because we don't talk about these matters. There are conversations about periods, and even graphic child birthing, but not the experience of fucking. I've already broken the privacy code of our friendship, which makes my heart gallop. "Do you think this is even real? Let's face it. I found a malady on the internet and diagnosed myself."

"It doesn't matter if we've heard of it," Gayle informs me. "The important thing is that you're open with your husband."

Gayle is always right.

✳

"Listen," I say to Kurt the moment I return from the restaurant.

"Listen," he repeats from his large desk in our teeny living room. He's updating his classical music blog, another of his erudite passions.

I position myself on the sofa behind him, waiting for my chance. "I have to talk to you about something," I say into the back of his chair, which happens to be shaped like a heart.

"Sure," he responds automatically.

"Can we do that?"

"Sure."

He's still contemplating his monitor, enraptured by a composer I can't identify. If he turned around, I wouldn't have his full focus. I've discovered that about him. I speculate this night is not ideal.

"I'm going to floss," I mumble.

"Floss," I think he says.

I get right into bed, pulling the duvet up to my neck. On a crisp white background is a tangle of red plants that tonight are just too chaotic. I close my eyes.

I doze. Suddenly, my spouse is standing there. He looks skinny, wearing only a T-shirt and underwear. Vulnerable—like me.

"I have to talk to you about something," I blurt out.

"What's wrong?" He has frozen mid-stance.

"I have this thing."

"A thing?"

"With my vagina."

"An infection?" he asks loudly.

Why do men think this is the only trouble down south? I make clear that no, this is different. Then I grab my laptop from the living room, bringing it to bed. Kurt shifts his weight from leg to leg while I try to locate the right URL. He keeps coming back to yeasty, itchy concepts. "Are you sure it's not an infection?"

"Here, I'll show you," I say, finding the vaginismus site. "Just come here." I pat the blanket until he joins me. I hand him the computer.

While he reads, I bury myself in down feathers. I want them to cushion hardness I keep landing on, or will land on.

After a moment, Kurt takes a robust inhale, followed by an even more robust exhale: "You have this?"

"Yeah."

"But it says intercourse is impossible." He giggles a little. "Isn't that what we've been doing?"

"I know. There are different kinds of vaginismus. Read below where it talks about pain."

He can't find the place at first, which annoys me. And my pointing out where he should be reading annoys *him*. But then he's at the text. The minute he finishes, he turns to me with eyes so sad they feel like my child, or something I need to take care of for the rest of my life but don't know how.

"How long have you had this?" he asks slowly.

"Since the beginning. Maybe."

"Since we started *dating*?"

"No. Before that. I think I've always had it."

His hand reaches for mine. It feels a little cold. Once our fingers interlock, I'm thinking we might warm each other. "Why didn't you tell me?" he whispers.

"I don't know."

Not sure what else to convey, I wrap my limbs around my lover's skinny frame. He's lost weight in the last few months. I should have asked him about it. *Why didn't I ask him?* I keep hugging his skin, which smells like the pool where he swims after work. I love that pool smell, but I pull away.

"I want to buy the kit they talk about. Is that okay?"

"Of course. Whatever you need. We can do whatever you need."

Kurt repositions us with his butterfly-stroke arms. We are on our backs now, and a calf of his is over mine. Our fingers graze, my pointer caressing his thumb.

Later, in the dark, when I think he's already sleeping, he speaks into the ceiling, saying what he's probably been thinking all along: "Don't you think you should also see a doctor?"

Maybe my life could be simple like that.

I'll do whatever it takes to have my very own Vagina Christmas.

Tips for *Your* Pleasure Plan

Something to Try:

Using a single sheet of paper, divide your page into three columns. At the top of each column, write (respectively): Medical, Emotional, and Pleasure Education. Now, list your bedroom challenges, putting them into the column you think each item should belong to. Don't worry about being right or wrong, and don't be afraid of feeling "broken." Part of your journey will be shifting your thinking around brokenness. Rather than using it as a defective label—condemning your entire existence—you'll be using it diagnostically. If it's broken, there's a good likelihood it can be fixed!

Journal Prompts:

1. Are you *really* "broken," or do you have one or more physical issues that might respond to medical attention? Examples include painful intercourse, vaginal dryness, muted orgasm, etc.

   _____

   _____

   _____

2. Are you *really* "broken," or do you have one or more psychological/emotional issues that might respond to psychotherapy? Examples include self-blame, shame, trauma triggers, lack of attraction to a partner, etc.

   _____

   _____

   _____

3. Are you *really* "broken," or do you have one or more issues that might respond to better information about your sexual and erotic self? Examples include not knowing what arouses you or having difficulty talking to a partner about your needs.

   _____

   _____

   _____

3

The Vacuum

"Look at that nice scarf," says Dr. Graham, the gynecologist I've seen on and off for the past ten years. She's referring to a pink and orange pashmina wrapped around me. It supplements blue paper barely covering flesh in this subzero-degree room. I haven't clarified my visit yet; I'm just perched on her exam table while my doctor studies a laptop sitting on a sanitized white shelf. The walls behind it are the same color as my dressing gown, which smells like nothingness—or possibly alcohol wipes. Graham is clicking on the keyboard as she says, "Let's see, the last time you were here was..."

Remorse pulls tight the corset of my chest, but there's also pride under my shawl. I'm proud my family hated doctors. Fuck you, Mengele. But Dr. Graham is *not* a Nazi. I actually have to remind myself of this, though not quite explicitly. It's more like I need her to prove herself to me, after a decade of coming here—albeit sporadically. I want to put my faith in her, like that time she discovered a fibroid, which she expertly got rid of. She did it with such friendly competence. I've always admired her petite runner's physique (so fit), her long blond hair (so shiny), her soft Long Island accent (so high-end shopping mall, so Lord & Taylor). Now she is washing her hands.

"Wait," I say, liberating an arm from under my scarf so I can use it as a stop sign. "Before you start, I think I have vaginismus. Do you know what that is?"

"Yes, I do." It comes out singsongy, which is nonetheless reassuring. Someone, besides me and the people on the vaginismus website, has heard of this ailment.

"Let me examine you, and at the end, I can test you for it."

There's a test?

A moment later, bony fingers make concentric circles on my breasts. Shit. I forgot this part, that it comes first. Before I can get clarity down yonder, I have to wander into another part of my minefield—my boob phobia. Like many women, I fear breast cancer. But *unlike* most women, I won't go for mammograms because of menacing Mengele, which rules out early detection, placing me at greater risk for . . . breast cancer. It's a conundrum that leaves me vulnerable in a way no pashmina can help. Presently, that fabric bunches around my throat.

As Graham continues her palpations, I think of the female cancers I could have. *Cervical. Ovarian. Uterine. Vaginal.* Aren't they all related? Breast and ovarian are. I should have seen Graham consistently. To hell with my dead mother and her murdered relatives. I should be getting mammograms. Then again, my mother never got these. I can't remember her ever seeing a gynecologist. She was fine. Everyone in my mother's house was fine—because of her secret remedies.

Whenever I got a cold, in lieu of drugs, and the people who prescribed them, Mom pumped me full of liquefied garlic, extracted from her Acme juicer. Then she'd haul out a thrift store Hoover. She used this to administer her prized respiratory remedy. In a stained housedress, with a forehead creased in concentration, my mother vacuumed my nose.

It was a final mucus solution she stumbled upon after the war. Settled safely in New York, my mom got a job in a bra factory, a place that was dreadful for her allergies. At Auschwitz, she'd also labored in a factory, sewing buttons on Nazi uniforms. She tried her best not to sneeze in that filthy barrack as they sent sick prisoners to the gas chamber.

Maybe she wanted to believe American doctors were different. She certainly wanted to keep her job. Allergies turning to asthma, Mom found an ENT specialist. This man with shiny shoes owned a suction device that extracted the "gunk" from her sinuses. Was it just her imagination, or did it resemble the canister contraption she used on her rugs?

After he was done treating my mother, the doctor smiled. His teeth were also shiny and expensive. He wanted to know how she felt.

"Good," she said to this man. *Shyster*, she said to herself. In other words, this guy was a thief, charging her for something she could do at home.

By the time I came along, Harriet Zam had perfected her technique. Step One took place in our kitchen pantry, which stank of rotting fruits and vegetables because Mom always bought too much food. (The rest of the house was also deeply dirty. And there were roaches, though strangely not in the pantry.) Anyway, the pantry is where she kept our thrift-store vacuum. For Step Two, she'd drag it into our purple living room, twisting off the long, metal pole and its carpet sweeping attachment; this freed the snaky hose. Step Three was offering it to me so I could place the metal base against my most clogged nostril. Step Four? Mom flipped the switch.

Every time I see that Mucinex commercial where anthropomorphized snot is drawn out of someone's sinuses, I smile because vacuuming your nose works just like this—only better. I love how DIY Mom was. I'm especially nostalgic for how she monitored phlegm levels, by yelling over the roar of the motor.

"Say 'Mommy,'" she'd scream, her face perspiring, her black kinky hair shooting out erratically.

"Mommy," I'd repeat as forcefully as the mucus would allow.

"You're still congested. I can hear it."

This went back and forth.

"Mommy."

"Say 'Mommy.'"

"Mommy."

"Say 'Mommy.'"

"Mommy."

"Say 'Mommy.'"

"Mommy! Mommy! Mommy!"

I should have lasting damage. But I don't have lasting damage. My nose is terrific.

According to Dr. Graham, who is finishing up her breast exam, my bosom is terrific too. "Well, I don't feel anything suspicious," she tells me.

See? Who needs doctors?

"Do you mind scooting down?" Graham asks, even though I have already engaged with this task. I slip my bare feet into her stirrups. She smears her finger with K-Y Jelly.

Me. I need a doctor.

Inside, my doc presses into delicate areas, wanting to know if anything she's doing causes pain. I say, "No," because I assume she's talking about extreme pain. *I don't know if my discomfort, current or otherwise, is extreme.*

"I have pain with intercourse," I exclaim. The phrase makes my mouth feel weird, like I was just chewing on a penny. *I have pain with intercourse.* "I'd just like you to get a full picture," I add, stroking my temples repetitively because her finger is being replaced by a speculum.

"Let me take a peek," she responds, followed by the inevitable: "Can you relax your legs a little?"

In the years since my first pelvic exam, I've gotten better (though not great) at knee opening. Does it hurt as much as the first time? You bet. At least I know what to expect, so it doesn't fog my wits.

In fact, despite the sharp pinching, my brain is lucid, more lucid than ever, given the circumstances. Questions rush into my brain, from dark recesses of denial and shame. I've never said these out loud—to Gayle, or Stacey, or my other friends. I certainly never talked to my mom about sex, not the mechanics, not anything beyond passion discussions. Who would have taught her proper anatomy, anyway? Her own mother was murdered when Mom was thirteen, and the family had been extremely religious. When my mother was sent to Auschwitz and made to strip in front of Nazi officers, she fainted from the shock of having men view her body.

I never talked about this level of detail with anyone. Perhaps that's why, now, my skull is crowded with thoughts that need to come out. "From what I read, vaginismus is just an entry issue. But I have other pain too. Do you know what might be causing that?"

"Let me see from the examination," she says.

"Because sometimes it seems like he's hitting the cervix. Is that normal?"

"I wouldn't say normal," replies the head poking out from between my legs.

"Oh…is it…do you think it's a position thing? Or is it something else?"

"These are good questions," says my gyno without her comforting singsong. "But it's difficult for me to answer while examining you. Why don't we talk when I'm done?"

Soon after, she performs the famous test. I think it's a Q-tip, but it feels like a hammer banging on the walls of my canal as if she's putting up pictures. Maybe some Georgia O'Keefe prints.

"Well, it looks like you *do* have vaginismus," my practitioner declares, taking off her rubber gloves.

Wow. This is real.

Still, is that the extent? She never addressed my other inquiry. As Graham leaves me alone to dress, I refuse to put on my outer layer, hopping back up on the table. I still need to know about thrusting, and burning, and pulling, and all the cervical stuff I was trying to get her to talk about.

The moment she reenters, I bombard her with a basic frame I think will put everything in perspective. "I think I need more information. I mean, if you read about sex, it says the vagina is supposed to expand ten inches. But unless a penis is ten inches, why would it hit the cervix?"

"It's not supposed to hit the cervix!" she says, with her attractive chin jutting forward at me. "It's supposed to go in the fornix."

I have no idea what a fornix is. I don't even get this word right. I'm convinced she just said *phonics.*

Put the penis in the phonics is what I hear as she points to a poster of the female reproductive system. Apparently, I'm using my hooha wrong.

I want to trust her, like that time with the fibroid. But as she goes through the parts—vagina, cervix, uterus—she's talking too fast, even for a New Yorker. I get the impression her medical school never ran courses like *Intro to Fucking for Physicians.*

My hands in my lap clench themselves into fists. Not out of anger. It's more like a way to reset. "I think what I'm trying to understand is what goes on during intercourse. I just need basic information."

Graham smiles at me with compassion, but then her eyes, which have been blinking every millisecond, flick to her dainty leather watch. "Why don't you make another appointment and we can just talk?"

"I'm sorry."

"No, *I'm* sorry. I'd like ... there's only so much time for each patient."

"I know. I know. I'm sorry," I mumble, wrapping the pashmina around my neck three times, though the weather that day is mild.

Before I go, Graham tells me to purchase something she calls genital weights. I picture tiny dumbbells, like what a squirrel might use to take off those extra acorn pounds. I'm instructed to work out with these every day, to strengthen my pelvic floor—precisely what the dilators are designed for.

"You don't think I should get dilators?"

"No, weights are better for this." She gives me a piece of paper with the name of a medical supplier.

Leaving her office, I wonder how many people are making a fortune off the vagina—having it suck up weights and speculums, and glass dildos and ridged vibrations. Everything you put near it. How many are making billions off our little vacuums? Suddenly, I feel like crying, which is ludicrous. I got what I came for. A validated disorder. A cure. At least for part of my problem. There's no reason to feel battered, especially after encountering enchantment, right outside the office.

A fifty-something pair—a man and woman—is standing there like a mirror image of me and Kurt. My heart starts squealing: *Hey, he's supporting her healing, just like my guy is supporting mine.*

I'm confident that Kurt would have been here too if I'd requested that of him. I didn't because attending to my lady parts—their function and lack thereof—has always seemed a solitary endeavor. I'm happy my husband's emotional double is here. Resembling George Clooney in a green ski jacket, his lined mouth and narrowed brow say: *I am a concerned and caring spouse.*

Observing more closely the recipient of his love, I see she's been sobbing—expressing *my* emotion. It's like one of those films where a Parisian couple wanders into a park while a puppet show is in progress. Serendipitously, the puppets act out the scenario the lovers are going through.

After watching a tad more of their drama (the man puts his arm around her hunched shoulders) I feel slapped across the face—by recognition. She's just been given a diagnosis. A terrible diagnosis. By Dr. Graham.

I zoom away from that death house as quickly as I can.

It takes me months to order the weights. I can't find the paper, which simply vanishes. To get a replacement, I just have to contact Graham, which I should do anyway to set up another appointment. To talk, only to talk. But I'm scared she'll humiliate me again.

"You said you were working on this," says Kurt about once a week, usually right after I've refused physical intimacy, again.

"I *am* working on it," I respond.

"Are you?"

"Yes."

"I thought you were going to get that kit."

"I know. But my doctor doesn't think it's a good idea. She wants me to get weights."

"So get the weights!"

"I can't find the paper! I'm going to look for it. I promise."

These arguments always lead to a night of lovemaking. Coitus without complaint. The sensation is like being punched on the inside like there is acid on my guy's member. It seems like progress, though, because unlike before, I can at least name the pain. But I'm having trouble imagining sex without it. I don't possess that kind of imagination. Sometimes, I chastise myself—*What's wrong with me? Why can't I get my fuck ducks in a row?*

Four months after seeing Graham, I chance upon the paper she handed me that day—buried in a file I never go into called "Health."

On the day the weights arrive, I rip open the box and find a white, plastic, four-inch bullet. There are three metal discs in the box too. These resemble the washers I've seen mechanical people (not me) replace on a faucet. The glossy, overly concise directions say I'm supposed to place the washers inside the bullet for extra ounces.

Unscrewing the cylinder is rather easy, as is adding the weight (I choose the lightest). On penetration, cold plastic hits the same genital doorway encountered by Jeremy, and everyone else who, over the years, has come a-knockin'. The little manual doesn't mention this dilemma. In fact, it recommends that after insertion I go outside and start "jogging."

Do these people have any knowledge at all about a woman's insides?

Surprisingly, I *do* push the weight in, a little, and I can stand in the living room with the bullet lodged in the vestibule, provided I jam my thighs together. It feels like I've been shot in my soft center.

When I remove this intruder, I am flooded with a long breath of gratitude. It awakens wild yet calm determination.

I don't want vaginal weights.

I don't want dilators.

I don't want tampons.

I don't want K-Y Jelly.

I don't want Q-tips.

I don't want fingers.

I don't want cock.

I don't want anything, anything inside me.

Tips for *Your* Pleasure Plan

Something to Try:

If you've not already brought up your problem(s) with a medical provider, try asking about it at your next appointment. Tell your practitioner, in advance, that you'll be asking a lot of questions. This person might postpone the exam itself, allowing you to just ask questions. Pay attention to your gut during this conversation. Trust your instincts about whether you are getting all the information you need, or whether you need to discover other resources and guidance. For a list of questions you might ask your doctor, see my website and blog.

Journal Prompts:

1. Are you comfortable talking to your gynecologist, urologist, therapist, or any other practitioner you might talk to about sex? If not, do you know where to look to find someone you're more comfortable with? See the Recommended Resources section in the Appendix for tips on how to find doctors and therapists with extensive training in sexual health and healing.

   _____

   _____

   _____

2. Is there someone in your orbit—a person with compassion and good information—with whom you might seek counsel regarding your sexual health?

   _____

   _____

   _____

4

A Plan

Kurt's in the kitchen, slamming cabinets. Pots. Pans. From my post in the next room—our pink sofa, watching the evening news—I smell the tomato-garlic of his creation: *Arrabiata*, an Italian dish that translates as "angry pasta." Have these noodles taken over his mood? More likely, it's the conversation we had earlier when I'd just returned home from teaching yoga.

He said: "You wouldn't want to give me a BJ, would you?"

And I said: "I'm so bloated." Then I went on and on about the afternoon croissant still stuck in my belly.

Eight months after our honeymoon, five months after stuffing those vaginal weights in a drawer, I still don't want physical intimacy—of any kind. I used to give in but now rely on a vast array of maladies: distention from naughty foods, post-dinner fatigue, constipation crabbiness, and chronic itchy-leg syndrome.

My first therapist, Maria, told me years ago, "Don't ever have sex if you don't want to. It will set back your recovery." I ignored her for the most part. But now that I've gotten closer to the source of my problems, I feel like respecting my desires. The aspiration from my honeymoon—moving beyond sex malaise—has been subsumed by wanting to pay attention. To me. I can't explain this to Kurt, though, because I fear he's going to get mad. And see? He is mad. But who can blame him for frustration?

As I try to watch television, my nostrils flaring, I realize I blame him. Or, more to the point, I frame him—as a child. *He's such a baby*, I think, turning my head toward the clamor of his cookery. A three-gallon cauldron is being maneuvered into our puny sink; he's filling it with water. Knowing his recipe, I can place the other scents and sounds: kale in one pan, sauce in another, plus the big bowl for salad. Since he's doing the meal prep, I'll need to clean this mess. It's a fair arrangement, of course it is. But tonight, his culinary expanse seems vengeful, juvenile.

"Are you mad at me?" I throw my voice into the hallway connecting the living room to our galley kitchen, which is minuscule.

"I'm not angry," Kurt shouts back. "But can you set the table?"

"Did you put the pasta in yet?" It's a rhetorical question because he just put the water on. I still have twenty minutes, at least, until it's ready. *Why am I always on his schedule?* "I'll set it later," I tell him.

"Can you please set the table?" he insists after making his way to the hallway so he can see me.

"Stop yelling at me!" I yell back.

This is the raised-voice way we talk to each other now, especially after a coded, or explicit, discussion about nooky. Other times, in lieu of this tension, there are formal tones like what we employ once the meal is served.

"Do you mind passing the greens?"

"Here you go."

It's like we're distant cousins meeting for the first time at a Bar Mitzvah. Now we're stuck sitting next to each other all night.

In between bites and sparse dialogue, I swivel my chair to watch

60 Minutes. Leslie Stahl is on. Her ruby lipstick makes me think of the fellatio I just refused. Surely, with her busy schedule, she must run into a similar dilemma—not being in the mood because she's narcoleptic or irregular from constant travel. But unlike me, she seems like a lovely person who'd oblige her husband. I used to perform without issue too, particularly when it got me out of penis-in-vagina action. But in the last few months, fellating without enthusiasm has seemed wrong. Maybe Leslie can go down on her man with ambivalence because she doesn't share my history. She doesn't need to explore celibacy the way I do.

Celibacy.

The word hovers above, like a halo. If I'm honest with myself, that's what I'm craving, or even pushing for here. Not directly though. Once upon a time, I was more direct.

When I was twenty-seven, I spent almost a year without sexual engagement of any kind. The idea came to me spontaneously after a freakish occurrence—I blacked out during sex. The moment before I'd been making love with my boyfriend Farez at a bed-and-breakfast in Pennsylvania. We'd woken up and immediately started fooling around. As he mounted me, I gazed out a window overlooking a rainbow of azaleas on the back patio. Beyond that was a luxurious forest. His maneuvers hurt me, but not uniquely. I remember inhaling the scent of the thin, patchwork comforter. It smelled like laundry detergent, a little floral and sweet. Then I was gone.

It's hard to say where I traveled to, how I got there, or how long I stayed. I was cocooned in darkness, outside space and time. On the periphery, images were present but they didn't touch my senses— viscous honey, an underground passage, a sewer permeated with sticky, thick honey.

"Where did you go?" is the phrase that brought me back. Farez was staring at me, and I noticed his sharp Lebanese features were softened.

"I don't know," was all I came up with. I knew I'd left the room and that I hadn't fallen asleep. It must have been dissociation. My new therapist, Maria, taught me this word after I talked to her about zoning out while fornicating—thinking about patent leather shoes I might acquire, for instance. But nothing like this had ever happened before. My attention still outside the window, I was hoping the array of flowers would throw me some language. "I don't know where I was," I continued. "But..."

Farez was sitting up, hairy legs crossed in front of him. He took my hand, which was limp.

My whole body was a weak sack of skin, but inside a dynamic pump pushed up a message from my soul. The whole situation was so strange; I didn't take time to apply a filter. I let the words forcefully exit my lips, "I don't want to be having sex right now."

My boyfriend peered into my face thoughtfully, "That's okay. We don't have to finish."

"No," I said with more volume, though I had no idea where this certitude was coming from. "I'm not talking about today. I mean all the time. I feel like I'm not meant to be having sex right now."

Farez and I broke up instantly.

He told me he couldn't be in a relationship that wasn't physically intimate because "I am a very sexual person." I don't recall begrudging him. I was busy figuring out, excitedly, how I might become a *non*sexual person. It wasn't just the acts. I would escape panic when a testosterone person expressed interest—or didn't. I'd be liberated from the gamut.

After that day, I deliberately began spending time with male friends, to see how it worked. With a couple of them, there had been mild, lopsided crushes—from him to me or me to him. But in my new abstinence only program, palpitations were deleted from our bond. I simply refused to think of these dudes romantically, and I was explicit: bed was not an option. All of a sudden, I didn't hate them. It was a wild revelation. *Had I always loathed this gender?* Yes! What's more, I'd been secretly harboring contempt.

Now, guys were great. I couldn't get over how adorable I found their quirks: the nervous wince when they touched their bald spots; their witty disdain for alpha assholes, even though they claimed they never gossiped; the drunken sighs of alpha assholes, who'd talk low in dive bars, but not lasciviously (not with me), confessing the exact same story about *her*, the only woman he ever loved, but she was troubled and fled the country, leaving him unable to love another, and that was fourteen years ago.

What a fabulous chunk of humanity these penis owners were.

And what a heavenly year.

Unfortunately, it came to an end, abruptly, when an old flame came to town. Tom, a tender horticulturist, was the first man to ever notice I never climaxed. I'd been sleeping with dudes for ten years at that point and not one of them had ever inquired into my peak experience. For the three months Tom and I dated, before he relocated to another state, he took it upon himself to reform my situation—to no avail. He was back in New York for a mutual friend's party, where I ran into him. At 3 AM, I was woken by his call.

I let him come by.

I let him deliver me to a morass of emotions I still wasn't able to navigate, even with my experiment.

Twenty years later, lounging on the couch with my husband, while watching the last chunk of *60 Minutes*, I ask myself, *Is male sexual energy any less scary or perplexing? Am I more capable of solving mysteries woven into my labia and soul?*

I study Kurt, who's currently snoring with his feet upon the coffee table. When he fell asleep, he crossed his arms over his chest as if he were a kid imitating a corpse. He seems so harmless. My heart is achy with my failure to be intimate. Yet, seeing him like this sends my wits off a cliff.

What if he *were* to die? He's eight years older than me, getting close to sixty. My mother died in her sixties of a heart attack. For a second, I let my imagination journey to an alternate universe where my husband no longer exists. On this alternate planet, I'm alone in this apartment. There's no amazing tomato sauce wafting through the air, no whiff of chlorine on a hearty man's skin. But there *is* more oxygen. My lungs take in this pretend extra gas.

It smells like freedom.

With Godspeed, I shut down the fantasy, loudly closing the coffin in my mind. I mean, opening it! I flagellate myself immediately. *How can you even hope for such a thing? What kind of horrible monster are you? How could you think to hurt this amazing person? How could you wish to be alone?*

The next time Kurt and I make love, which is the next night—my suggestion out of guilt and angst—I place a journal near the bed. It's a blank book with red flowers on the cover, where I intend to record what the hell's going on. Part of my resistance to relations, I'm grasping, is that I'm overwhelmed by my vagina. What I tried explaining to Dr. Graham, my gynecologist, is that I *don't* just have vaginismus, which is an entry issue. I have other kinds of pain too. And everything is getting worse. *Why is it getting worse?* If I want to save my marriage, which I do—I absolutely do—I need clarity here.

That's why as my guy and I comingle, I choose a straddling top position where there's better control. Here's what I decode while fucking: *The whole front side of the vagina ... or you could call it the top ... no, it's the front ... the front wall ... it's irritated. Like a ... sheet.* A *sheet of irritation.* That's how I'm going to describe it later in my bedside book, which I have dubbed my Screw Journal.

Moving my sheath slowly up and down the shaft, I stay in literary mode. *Sheet of irritation* is going to be joined by ... *general inflammation,* and also ... *scabs inside my vagina.* Or, *scabs in the corners,* a phrase that makes no sense, so I chuckle.

"What's funny?" asks my lover as his eyes go from blue to gray. With his sweaty hair standing straight up, he looks like a person you'd never suspect to be violent until he is. Gentle Kurt has never displayed tendencies of this nature. But my dad wasn't violent either—except perhaps he was, according to my mom those times she called the cops. What about the Nazis who murdered my family? Most of them, at home, were probably the sweetest of teddy bear papas.

"Nothing is funny," I tell my man. Then I paste on a mask of enjoyment—smiley half-open lips and sultry half-closed eyes. For inspiration, I lift my gaze to a giant black-and-white photo above our headboard. A young starlet from the fifties stands in front of a theater in a swan-like gown that gathers in the rear. Men halt to behold her.

I stay like this a long time, circling my hips, so I can nail words into my skull: *soreness ... inflammation ... sharp objects ramming into hip joints ... stomach blows ... shooting leg pain ... being sewn shut ... being ripped open ... like scabs ripped away ... tearing tissues ...*

Ripping, tearing tissues ...

I can't bear it anymore. But I don't stop.

How else will he get enough friction?

For thirty years, I've been giving men friction.

For thirty years, I've been giving men friction will definitely make it into my Screw Journal. But right now I want to sob with big heaving waves. My whole being contracts to avoid this. It's the wrong kind of contraction. I strap down my animal sadness so I don't saturate the bed with the wrong kind of moisture.

And yet, tears do fall.

"Are you crying?" Kurt has stopped moving—thank God. He's staring at me.

"It's okay," I whisper.

"It's not okay." He withdraws. He's facing me now on his side, close to my body. Too close. He moves strands of my hair so they're not blocking my face. "What is it?" he wants to know. "Did I force you? Do you feel like I forced you?"

"No." I am shaking my head as more sorrow rises up and out of my squeezed tight eyes.

"I'm so sorry," he says without knowing what he did. He pulls me to his chest. But I turn myself around so he's spooning me. I assure him, it was some "old shit" that came up for me. Then I wait for him to sleep. The tears have stopped by this point. I need my eyes for other activities. I stare into blackness, summoning illumination—a lit up idea. Even just a sliver. Nothing appears. The truth is, Kurt is not the baby. I am.

But it's time to grow up because I *do* know what I want here. I want to be more than just a friction machine. I really do. I just don't know how to make that happen.

Then I get the call.

A few days later a Jewish theater is on the line, a missive totally unrelated to my marriage. Yet, it's the kind of random event that could change the course of a person's life, if she let it.

The person ringing me up is a fabulous director named Shirley, who knows about my six one-person plays. She directed my most recent, and I love her work. Her voice through my receiver says her theater, a small-but-prominent venue, wants to commission me to create a new piece. I can write about anything I want.

On the spot, I decide I'm going to write about my carnal disabilities, overcoming them. What most appeals to me about this endeavor is the deadline. In the six months they give me to whip up this drama, launching this summer—from August 2011 until January 2012—I'll have to figure out how to rise above my past and become a sexual person. They'll help me, however, through regular meetings focused on the structure of my play. This package of goodies sets off pounding in my torso, like terror and titillation as a single emotion.

Shirley tells me I'll be presenting my material in front of a live audience because the deal includes a reading. "Do you really want to do that?" she asks. Nervous giggles add staccato height to her deep voice.

"I do." It comes out resolute, surprisingly.

"Well, okay, then," says my director, who adds after a brief pause, "what's not to love?"

Her phrase reminds me that the Jewish theater—and now my curative project—have their roots in vaudeville.

After I get off the phone, I search for my Screw Journal. Once it's in my hands, I spontaneously compose a list:

- Hypnotist
- Sex Therapist
- EMDR
- Emotional Freedom Technique

- Tantrika
- Workshop for Couples
- Trauma Therapist

My thinking is that I'll use the half-year of writing time to see a panoply of experts who might shed light on my issues and even cure me. I'll document my sessions and what they teach me, here, in this diary, which will become the foundation for my play. I gape at the practitioners I just wrote down.

They're based on what I know, that is, what I've gleaned the last twenty years being in therapy. (As recently as a few months back, I was seeing a psychologist named Karen. I stopped with her because she didn't realize what vaginismus was.) What I know is trauma. But not just as a patient. Trauma infuses all three branches of my career: story-telling projects with varied populations, including soldiers returning from Iraq, teens from the Middle East, and women at a rape crisis center; the K-12 drama lessons I do, which are trauma-informed; and teaching yoga, which includes working with abuse survivors.

Ultimately, though, the experts I've jotted down are based on what I *don't* know. Despite this work on myself, and experience in recovery arenas, I still can't figure out my history. I mean, what is the source of my sexlessness? Is it molestation events locked in my body? Ignorance about female eroticism and mechanics? Lack of information about matrimony and the way it alters intimacy? Marriage surely alters sex. Everybody says. But how? Which of these is the actual springboard? I think it's all of the above. I certainly feel broken in each of these areas. The only way I'll get better is by approaching my healing from multiple perspectives.

Seven.

Seven varied professionals seem perfect. *Seven Habits of Highly Effective People.* Seven Wonders of the World. Seven chakras, too. My favorite aspect of teaching yoga is talking about these esoteric wheels of energy. I think of their alignment right then, to settle the handball bouncing in my gut, because . . . it begins dawning on me what I've just committed to. I'm not just making a freakin' list. I'm going to actually visit these healers, who mostly terrify me. Sex therapy? Yikes. Plus, I have to resolve my *forty-year* trauma within months! And then there's the part about performing my vag-woes on the stage, in front of hundreds of people. My whole body feels like it's bouncing now, in a jeep, in a war zone.

As a touchstone, I call my best friend, Wendy. She's a brilliant novelist and the most sensible person I know. While my tendency is to reach for billowy shirts on Visa, Wendy holds firmly to her pen. Consequently, she's published three excellent books. Upon hearing my idea, Wendy says: "You're an artist. Art is how you process things."

Her validation helps me understand my own motives. "It's the only place I believe in myself," I confess while biting a piece of my hair. Then, I talk about decades of honing faith that order will arise from creative chaos. Since getting my B.A. in Theatre from Brooklyn College, I've done it a million times: strategizing, organizing, meeting deadlines, and finally delivering something substantial at the end of a theatrical process.

Wendy assists me in thinking through how I'm going to finance this initiative, which seems daunting at first. She helps me realize that most of the professionals I'd like to see should be covered by my health insurance, which is great at reimbursing for therapy. Regarding other expenses, the theater will give me a little money. But I'll need to save up from my multiple jobs. No debt. My best friend and I agree on that. "You've got this," she says as my heart travels across hundreds of miles to hug her.

Right after this conversation, I go back to my list and write above it *The Plan*. I want a name capturing the doable, the concrete. But considering this nomenclature, I decide to spice it up with more literary panache. I cross out *The Plan* and write *The Pleasure Plan*.

Then I close this diary and peer at the cover. Though I've been unofficially calling this my Screw Journal, I never wrote it anywhere on the journal itself. I now give this book an official name. On the front cover, with a black Sharpie, in big cursive letters, I write *The Pleasure Plan*.

In other words, *The Pleasure Plan* is not just my list or notes regarding practitioners I'll try. Nor is it just a draft of my play. It's all of these. My whole immense endeavor. My very own experiment in healing.

Kurt needs to know about this. Indeed. Luckily, he likes to iron, a menial task not too demanding but absorbing enough. This is particularly true since our apartment is teeny, inspiring him to rig our dining room table as an ironing board; it's tricky making this work. I've discovered if I'm embarrassed discussing a topic with my husband—like plump credit card balances—ironing is a good time to talk. In essence, he's not one hundred percent listening. Fresh off the phone, I stand next to his de-wrinkling.

"So, I think I know what I'm going to write about," I say after telling him about the commission, which he's excited about. My feet, throughout, are pointing and flexing, like I'm a ballerina. It's a nervous habit I acquired after my mom signed me up for ballet at the Little Theater School when I was six. Call it confidence through grace. "I think it's going to be about my sex problems." I continue, "*Our* sex problems."

"What do you mean?" Kurt asks as his shoulders hike.

"That didn't come out right," I reply. "I want to write about healing from my trauma. I mean, getting better."

He doesn't say anything, but the iron steams, like a sigh. Kurt is the only man I know who won't send his dress shirts to the cleaners. He says it's because it's more economical, but I suspect the real reason is that he doesn't want anyone to see his food stains and underarm discoloration.

"What do you think?" I repeat in case he didn't hear me. Apparently, he did.

"To me," he begins, "it sounds like you're trying to relive your trauma. Why would you want to go back there?"

"It's just a play," I throw at him, knowing it's not just a play. It's my only way of ever moving forward. "Listen, I need to do this. I'll let you read everything. Okay? You can approve everything."

He's silent again. I wait. I need his blessing. Kurt gets to the collar of his shirt before he replies, "I don't understand why *you* don't understand that some things are private."

He's right. I don't understand. Privacy is the garage where a four-year-old was exploited and damaged. Privacy is a penis getting hard in my hair as an old man made sure no one noticed. Privacy has stolen my life force. I thought *The Pleasure Plan* was about my marriage, and it is. But it's also about me. ME, no longer being small and stuck and tight and dead. It's about a pulsing power of aliveness that I'm missing.

I am determined to get it back.

Tips for *Your* Pleasure Plan

Something to Try:

Think of your healing as an experiment. All you'll need is a dedicated journal or computer file. Start making a list of what could possibly help your situation. In making this list, you're stimulating fresh thinking and summoning courage to try the unknown. For accountability, find a way to document your experiment—through a video, an Instagram series, a one-person play, a fictionalized story, a scrapbook, etc. You don't have to share this material with anyone. Or do share it! Either way, a physical manifestation will help you organize your journey and rise above it, where you might not feel as stuck.

Journal Prompts:

1. Where are you stuck in your sexual healing?

_____

_____

_____

2. Is there anyone who could help you proceed?

_____

_____

_____

3. Can you make a list of everyone you think could help you?

_____

_____

_____

4. Can you reach out to the first person on the list?

_____

_____

_____

Part 2
A Plan to Heal

5

My Vajahna Is Very Open, I Think

Now that I have *The Pleasure Plan* guiding me, mapping out my progress, and yanking me out of paralysis, I'm on the highway, traveling to the first person on my list—the hypnotist. This is not my initial visit though. At that session with Dr. Fay, mentioned previously, she wouldn't hypnotize me because she didn't think I was "a sexual person." I convinced her to see me again, anyway. But at my second appointment, she *still* wouldn't hypnotize me, claiming she had to get to know me better. Today, however, is the day. For this third meeting, Dr. Fay is finally going to put me in a trance.

Cruising the Beltway, connecting my DC home to her suburban Maryland office forty minutes away, I should be nervous, but I'm singing along to Led Zeppelin on the radio. Propulsive guitar makes me feel like I'm advancing. I am. I made this woman give me what I desire. It's not arbitrary. I always wanted to be hypnotized.

When I was a kid in the 1970s, autosuggestion was a popular Vegas act that found its way to the many televisions in our home. We had one in each room because Mom compulsively bought thrift shop clothes and appliances. She claimed if she stopped buying, she'd get sick. Our TVs frequently featured a mesmerizer overseeing a cute blond hugging a coworker after a guy in a tie acted like a chicken.

This is exactly the experience I yearn for. Not to become the chicken but to have another take control. I won't remember a thing as the brain whisperer swoops in and takes away my brokenness, like a tumor discovered in time. I'll simply wake up and it will be gone.

Or, at least my vaginismus will be gone. Hypnotherapy is a known remedy that doesn't involve intrusion like those horrid weights. Once I'm mended, the other practitioners can do their magic, addressing my *other* challenges—with libido, arousal, climax, and the gamut. I'm harmonizing with Robert Plant because pushing for this modality was right. It's the lynchpin to my plan's success.

Yet, suddenly my hands go sweaty on the steering wheel. It's sinking in. This is real hypnosis, not a Vegas act. Won't we venture into abuse? Dr. Fay told me several times she didn't think my past is related to current problems, so I wasn't thinking we'd go there. But what if buried memories come up anyway? Like many survivors, I recall my harm in fragments. Do I really need to know about other events? My recollections are bad enough.

They start now, staccato flashbacks. It's like my psyche is trying to protect me. If I can bring these up now I won't have to root around later, unearthing what I do not want to find. The pervert in the garage resembling Pope Benedict, he's a starring actor. I see him approach as I play in the street; I'm being undressed; he's taking me inside his house to meet his wife. Then another predator is in my cranium—because my block, unbelievably, had *two* pedophiles. Harvey is wobbling over, his gut hanging over his belt; he's rubbing up against my back as I toss a ball; a different time, he's asking me if I want to practice throwing. This predator morphs into a teenage boy my mother hired as a handyman; I'm on his lap; he's bouncing me on his hard penis; I partially understand he has a hard penis.

Getting out of my car in the hypnotist's parking lot, my legs feel like Jell-O. Not what I can buy today, but the stuff we ate in 1967.

"Why don't you sit, Hon?" Dr. Fay seems distracted as she stands facing a dark wood bookcase. She's searching for an item. I stand also in the center of her office, having just entered, thumbs hooked into the straps of my backpack like a student on her first day of school. I'm wondering if I should ask her to sidestep my history. I don't want to bring it up, though, giving her ideas.

"We'll get started in a moment," she announces without looking at me. Then she turns and smiles. "Have a seat," she says in her friendly Southern way.

When I do what she advises, on the ruby leather sofa, my thighs find each other like two anxious friends hugging.

"We'll start in just a minute," she reiterates as she pulls out books and rifles through them. A short while later, she exclaims, "I'm ready." She's holding a piece of letter-size printing paper that she strolls over to her plum velvet chair. Once she settles in, she leans forward and her smile drops. "Just so you know, I'll be planting images in your subconscious. But we will *not* be discussing your childhood. I do not think it's relevant."

"That's fine!" I say, but she doesn't hear me.

"I know *you* think it's relevant, but I do not. . . ."

"I agree," I assert. Then my legs unclench because, although I once worried this shrink might be incompetent, I've changed my mind. She's brilliant.

She looks the part too. Wire-frame readers have found their way to her face. She's a hot librarian in her tight, off-white slacks and silk cream shirt. Above the latter's pearly buttons, in her brain, is a card catalogue of eroticism she'll impart to my subconscious. I already feel prettier than when I walked in. But then something startles me.

It's right beside her, on the floor. Shaking himself out is a fluffy white dog that was absent the other times I came here. What's more, it's unmistakable: Dr. Fay is dressed similar to this animal. The same colors. Was it an accident?

"Okay," she says, still studying her paper. "I'd like you to lie down now."

I decide her outfit was an accident as I lean back in my own attire—black, wide-legged pants and a ribbed cotton tank. It's purposely almost pajamas. Somewhere, off in the distance, a bell jingles from a dog collar. I block it out, concentrating on the low vibration of her voice.

"Just breathe," says the vixen that will cure me. "Close your eyes."

I close my eyes.

"I'm going to relax you."

"I want to be relaxed," I tell her.

"Good," she replies. "I would like you to tense the toes of your right foot."

I comply.

"I would like you to release the toes of your right foot."

I comply.

"I would like you to tense the toes of your left foot."

I comply.

"I would like you to release the toes of your left foot."

I comply. But also peek. She's reading from her typed paper, which must be a script. I'm curious if she created this just for me, or if it's generic.

"I would like you to tense the calf of your right leg."

Yeah, I'm thinking it's generic, though I'm not sure I care. Look, even if she's not experienced, these are standard methods of producing tranquility. I use them with my yoga students all the time—because they work! As the hypnotist takes me through my whole body, I tense and release dutifully.

"Now repeat after me," she says, once this process is complete, "I am a very sexual person."

"I am a very sexual person," I parrot automatically.

"I love having sex with my husband," she says.

"I love having sex with my husband," I mimic. By now, I'm confused. Is this a trance state? I should ask. Rather than doing so, I cross and uncross my ankles, forcefully, to test if I'm unconscious. Obviously, I'm not. So now my entire being is tensing without the release part. I'm mad. But my unaltered state is only one grievance. Another is that I've already gone through this exercise—by myself.

At my second session with her, Dr. Fay gave me a handout on Cognitive Behavioral Therapy, or CBT, the kind of therapy she practices. It spoke of affirmations to rewire my brain. These could replace "limiting thoughts." Dr. Fay instructed me to record my voice on my iPhone, making sultry statements. In other words, she wanted me to talk dirty to myself. It seemed silly, but returning home, I locked myself in the bedroom where I improvised filth I hoped might make me wet. Then I went for a run.

As erotica seeped from earbuds into gray matter, I pounced on gray pavement until I reached a park. The trees there were shocking. They were so much greener than usual, and they were flirting. The trunks seemed...unabashed, calling attention to their girth. Branches were belly dancer arms, beckoning. Grass tickled my sneakers as I jogged. But it was colors I kept coming back to. They weren't just intense; they were immodest—emerald and amber, crimson and chestnut. Decadent nature was trying to get inside my skort. It was like fucking the entire planet.

I did similar orgy runs three times that week. At the end of those seven days, Kurt and I made love. I felt shifted—more beautiful than bloated. I kept touching my curls. My vagina, however, was straight up unresponsive. Like always. That was two days ago. I was hoping hypnosis would offer actual transformation.

I'm still hoping as Dr. Fay continues her randy phrases. I try reproducing her antebellum cadence.

She: "Mah vajahna is very open."

Me: "My vagina is very open." (My voice, however, sounds closed.)

She: "I do not have pain in my vajahna."

Me: "I do not have pain in my vagina." (A little more animated. Good.)

She: "My vajahna opens like a flahr."

Me. "My vagina opens like a flower." (I say this very slowly.)

I'm deliberate with energy and pace as we go on, but I'm skeptical any result can come of this encounter, especially in the remaining time. My mind wanders to her dog. What's *he* doing during these incantations? Does he have an erection? I hope so. I'll put it in my play. This whole experience, I'm beginning to think, is a joke that will make its way to my drama.

But then a funny thing happens on the way to the flahr.

I see it. The genital bloom the hypnotist has been touting. My consciousness is suddenly filled, to capacity, with a fuchsia orchid as audacious as the grass I played footsie with. The scene morphs. Now the orchid becomes purple like Dr. Fay's chair. Then it's an animated film, petals waving. The experience is like a daydream (I'm definitely not asleep). Or I'm swimming in imagination that may have powers. Can anatomy be renewed through artful invention? A sculptor with clay; perhaps a writer with her play. I am floating in this potential. But then I hear: "Let's come back to the present moment. I would like you to tense your right foot..."

Ah. It's over.

Dr. Fay grounds me again with her body scan. After, I'm sitting up as she burns me a CD.

"Should I listen to it every day?" I ask, gathering my belongings. I mention the original handout with affirmations. It stressed regularity.

"You *could* do it daily," says Dr. Fay walking me to the door. "Though probably? You don't need to." Holding out the disk, she adds: "This session should be enough."

It had better because I am never coming back here.

That night, I initiate thrusting to find out if anything took hold. Hubby doesn't complain. In fact, it makes him reconsider his objections to my project—and to the hypnotist herself. When I kept going back to her, he was suspicious: "Who *is* this woman?" Now he's elated she came into our life.

Under the covers, I join with Kurt as best I can. My bud is as tight as ever.

Post-lovemaking, curled on my side, I start hearing another kind of recording altogether. It's parental words stored in a microchip, maybe in my marrow. I hear my dad's voice with distinct Brooklyn vowels, "Lawra, you want my advice? I'll tell you right now. Don't want *anything*." I can see his long nose behind my eyes, a proboscis just like mine. I picture his pale skin from lounging in bed all day. "That way, if you get it, you'll be happy. And if you don't, you won't be disappointed."

It took me years to comprehend the truth of his proclamations. They were about his life—not mine. I'm not the person who went to Hollywood after the war trying to be an actor, only to come home defeated. I'm not the one who hated working the graveyard shift at the post office, who, by daylight, lay about in his undershorts, yelling at the television. I'm not the recluse whose only social activities were off-track betting and yearly vacations without wife and children. I'm not the patient who denied his degenerative disease even though he couldn't drive and had an unsteady gait.

Beginning around age twelve, I argued with him—without mentioning where I thought his negativity came from because saying so seemed cruel. Regardless, I fought him then. I fight him now: *That makes no sense, Dad. Everybody needs wishes. Everybody needs hope.*

When I'm done yelling at my father's ghost, I'm exhausted by righteousness, but then the tape plays, again, "Lawra, you want my advice? Don't want anything."

Dr. Fay is wrong.

A compact disk overlaying old thought patterns is not enough. Just like lascivious language in a pseudo-trance is inadequate. I need to go beyond my head and completely, fearlessly, look at my sick body—beyond my own denial. For that, I want to work with a brave heart who is unafraid to look.

I think I know exactly who that is.

Tips for *Your* Pleasure Plan

Something to Try:

Go out into nature and notice it—sex everywhere! Reproduction is busting a move via startling peonies, berry-rich bushes, frenetic fish, even ants crawling all over your picnic blanket. Allow yourself to soak in this force—life, giving rise to itself. Try imagining that you're a vital part of this perpetuating, creative, erotic planet. Notice . . .

Journal Prompts:

1. When do you feel most alive? Where are you when you feel this way? What are you doing? How does your body feel when you're most alive?

   _____

   _____

   _____

2. If you were on a treasure hunt for pleasure, where would you look?

   _____

   _____

   _____

6

The Mountain

I t's time to turn this over to God. By which I mean Goddess. The next morning, I go back to *The Pleasure Plan* journal. I press it hard against my torso, squishing my breasts—and the mighty beat behind them. A lady inside this book, on my list, is not afraid to peer at my nether region, and she'll do it in a holy manner. This person also knows how to remove demons she encounters. Am I talking about an exorcist? No. It's a Tantrika, an expert in sacred sensuality.

When I included a tantric mistress as part of my project, I did so because trauma, in many ways, is a state of disconnection. Spiritual professionals specialize in reconnection, don't they? That's why it's time to put down my journal and actually find a practitioner. Easy enough. I sit at my desk and google *Tantrika*.

The first hit is a superfit, fifty-ish woman with angular short, brown hair, like a twenties movie star. In one photo, she sits in a tropical Garden of Eden, on a rock, poised in meditation. All she has on is a diaphanous turquoise wrap. Her arms, athletic and well-shaped, are attached to long fingers. Testimonials on her site say things like: "The afternoon I spent with Francesca changed my life forever," and "Francesca took away my trauma with her touch."

Could I let this mystical woman touch me too?

Maybe it's simple: just as hands harmed me, hands are needed to heal me.

To find out, I have to leave the computer and pick up the phone. I mean it's only tantra. I love tantra, or what I memorized from my yoga teacher certification five years before. This ancient philosophy was developed and passed down by females for hundreds of years. Tantra harnesses erotic energy for transcendent connection—to a partner and also the divine. Rather than denying our physical experience in order to play with gods and goddesses, tantra wants us to embrace embodiment as a means of reaching beyond it.

Yes, contact with higher realms—man or woman in the sky, the Universe, or LIFE (her big-breasted self) is part of my recovery. With unfamiliar confidence, I know this to be true, though, how is still perplexing.

I pick up the telephone but don't dial. It's not just lack of clarity. My hand is shaky and my jaw feels locked. It's the same nervousness I felt when I used to lie to my mother about where I was going—so I could check out a synagogue.

Religion was shunned in our home. Before the war, Mom had been devoutly Jewish like her parents. When Hitler invaded Poland, she trusted that Yahweh would deliver her loved ones. But in the Lodz Ghetto, in Auschwitz, at Stutthoff (another concentration camp), Nazis killed her kin, including five members of her immediate family. Mom incrementally lost her faith. Ultimately, she felt duped.

On Saturdays and Sundays, my mother would give us her *own* sermons. We'd be running an errand, my brother and I in the back seat, when we'd happen upon a church, synagogue, or mosque. Pulling over, she'd point at those walking into houses of worship. "Look at those assholes," she'd shout at us. "They think God is going to save them." Then she'd scream through the glass: "GOD IS NOT GOING TO SAVE YOU!"

It wasn't until I moved out of my parents' house, at twenty-one, that I admitted to myself how spiritually curious I was. In my own apartment, I filled my bookshelves with books on Eastern philosophy, staying clear of Judaism, which was too loaded for me. Eventually, I turned to yoga, in text and practice.

This memory of my holy history, the arc of it, and the validation of my natural metaphysical interest help me finally dial the number displayed on the Tantrika's website, amidst those racy and calm photos. No one answers. Faced with her voicemail, I hang up. Deity? Diva? It doesn't matter. I'm still terrified of this woman and her see-through scarf. Perhaps I'm scared of how she might help me.

Then the phone rings.

"Allo?" says a foreign accent. Her web info said she was Italian. "Did you just call me?"

"Yes. Hi. My name is Laura."

"Hello Lauura," she says with earthy musically. Then her voice goes soprano and breathless. "Listen, I'm driving down a mountain in Maui, so we might get disconnected."

Shame flushes my cheeks because I've knocked at an inopportune moment. Her promise of elevation above my quivering body is my prayer though. I hurriedly detail my problems.

When I'm done, the Tantrika shouts her diagnosis from the mountain: "It sounds like a shrinking vagina."

A nervous laugh erupts in my throat because *shrinking vagina* is ridiculous. But so is the word *vaginismus*. I'm no longer dismissing the absurd. In fact, two of my friends—including my best buddy

Wendy—told me they think they also have vaginismus. Like me, they never had a name for extreme tightness. I've been helping them with my fledgling research.

There are so many questions I should ask Francesca right then, but only one pops out of me: "Is this something you treat?"

"Yes!" she answers. "Here's what I want you to do. When I return to New York, you must visit my studio with your husband and make love in front of me. In that way, anytime you feel pain, I can stop you. We need to figure it out, in the moment."

What she's saying makes perfect sense, but my viscera are trembling again.

"My husband will never go for this. Can't I see you by myself?"

"No. It won't work." I imagine her frowning, beautifully. "It's the only way."

I thank her and hang up. Then I stare out the window of the office nook in my living room. Above the desk is a vision board featuring dewy, successful women. I ignore it, fixating on what's in front of me: a gravel roof covering the lobby of my building, as well as the other half of this apartment complex. It's similar to most residences I've occupied in my adulthood—across the way, brick walls.

However, what if I'm done with thick, blocking brick?

When Kurt comes back from work, I follow him around the house. He's removing his jacket and tie. He's taking off his shoes. I work up the guts to say, "So, I had an interesting chat today. With a Tantrika."

"Tantrika, huh? Is that a woman who practices tantra?" He is getting into shorts and a T-shirt.

"You know everything, don't you?" I stir these words, seductively.

"Maybe. . ." He shows me his profile, nose lifted. A cartoon pose of pride, but he's beaming for real.

"Anyway," I continue, following him into the kitchen, where he, gratefully, stays put. "This woman, the Tantrika, she knows what's wrong with me." When I tell him about the shrinking vagina, he laughs so hard he almost spits out the hazelnuts he's munching on. It *is* hysterical. A joke. But when I get to the part about making love in front of her, I'm no longer laughing.

"What did you tell her?" he inquires.

"I said my husband would never do such a thing." I let the sentence linger like a bad smell I emitted. I should exit this room immediately, but I can't halt what's coming out of my mouth. "I mean, would you?"

"You're kidding, right?" He is no longer snacking.

I start persuading him to stick his dick inside me in front of a witness. My tongue feels swollen, but it needs to be said: "This woman *knows* how to help me."

"You really think that?" His voice is getting louder, "You think that?" Then he launches into a monologue about how *The Pleasure Plan* is warping my perceptions. It's not doing anything but digging up bad memories, which I am intentionally reliving, destructively.

"It's pathological," Kurt chants at least three times.

He's worried about me. He's worried about us.

Tips for *Your* Pleasure Plan

Something to Try:

> Make the call.

Journal Prompts:

1. What scares you when it comes to moving forward?

   _____

   _____

   _____

2. What scares you about *not* moving forward?

   _____

   _____

   _____

3. If you were to make one scary phone call pertaining to your sexual healing, whom would you call?

   _____

   _____

   _____

7

The Sex Brunch

I'm worried about us too. If I don't see the Tantrika, or the others on my list (who else is objectionable?), then my recovery map is useless. Then I'm right back where I started, immobilized in the mud.

Luckily, right after the Francesca call, and fight with Kurt, my friend Tamar and I meet for tea. I tell my pal everything. She tells *me*, for the first time, that she was assaulted in college. After knowing her for five years, after millions of heart-to-hearts about relationships, I'm surprised she never disclosed this. Tamar and I concur: women don't speak openly about our sexual histories. We're too ashamed. But, suddenly, my friend and I declare we'd like to fix that. Over cups of matcha, we decide to co-host a Sex Brunch three weeks hence. Her living room, three times the size of mine, will be the site.

Now nine giggly females, aged twenty-five to sixty-five, are about to share their fantasies, or their carnal complications, or *my* carnal complications; getting advice from other vagina-owners is definitely my agenda here. Standing before this bevy of brains I begin, "Welcome to what I hope will be the first of many Sex Brunches."

Then I mention the cards. Each woman is to write questions on supplied index cards, dropping them, once complete, in a small wicker basket, which I wave in the air. "In this way, we can elicit assistance anonymously," I impart to everyone. "In case anyone is shy, like me." To encourage participation, I pass around the cards and pens. Then I write my own queries. They read:

1. When you don't want to be physically intimate, what are the reasons?
2. Does anyone else have painful penetration? If so, what are some remedies?

After writing this second entry on my card, I pause. I'm not sure if I should seek additional counsel, based on an event that took place between tea with Tamar and today. I'm not sure if I should talk about the bomb that Kurt dropped six days ago.

"Listen, I have something to tell you," he said, right as we sat down for breakfast. He didn't say anything else though. He just played with the buttons on his flannel pajamas, staring down at the eggs I had made him. Then it came out. "I cheated on you," he said.

After absorbing this sentence, all I could hear were my cells multiplying. They were extremely loud, making it impossible to concentrate on anything else. Still, I managed to produce a word: "When?"

"2007," he said.

I left the cells alone to begin doing math. The year 2007 started a few months after we met—but two years *before* we got married. I took a deep breath. *He didn't break our vows.* More air going in and out. *He didn't break our vows.*

Inspecting my eyes the whole time, my spouse relayed the details of a beer-soaked tryst at a conference. In Vegas, for heaven's sake.

I needed more details. Questions shot out of me like arrows.

"*Which* conference?"

One of the ethics events he attends—oh, the irony.

"Who was she?"

Someone doing like-minded work at a different organization, in a different city.

"Did you use a condom?"

Yes!

"Has it happened since?"

No!

What I didn't ask him was *why*.

It stumbled out anyway, "We had just started dating, and ... I wasn't used to being hit on. . . . I think I was just curious."

"You were curious," I echoed. Undoubtedly, he was *curious* about what it might be like to not penetrate a chastity belt. Why wouldn't he want to be free from the tethers of pedophilia? However, my past was not to blame here. *He* was the one who betrayed *me*. "So why are you telling me this now, five years later?" I asked as if I had fallen asleep only to wake up with a jolt and a whole new probe.

Kurt's blue eyes blew up into what you might find on a frightened beast. He revealed that the impetus for his confession, shockingly, was *The Pleasure Plan*. "Believe me; this has been eating at me. I didn't know how to tell you. But now that we ... We're being honest with each other, right?"

"Uh-huh," I mumbled. Then I tried to eat my eggs, but the floorboards underneath my feet rumbled like a subway runs under my building. It doesn't. I couldn't stop thinking: *What else will this Pleasure Plan reveal? Has he told me everything about the affair? Are there others?* I couldn't stop thinking about another man in my life that had wandered—my father.

Before they got married, Mom pleaded with Dad to leave other women alone. They wed with a promise that he would. But after the wedding, he continued messing around, even after my brother and I came along. I think Mom left the house sometimes so my father could screw one of her friends. My mother only hinted at these crimes, but it was enough to further destabilize my home.

"It's fine. Let's eat," I finally said to Kurt, ending this unpleasant discussion. I reasoned: if he'd waited five years to disclose, I might never have to think about this again.

At the Sex Brunch, I do think about it, of course, because here would be a natural place to get guidance. Yet, how might asking these ladies help? Also, I don't want others to think badly of my guy. Mostly though, I'm wondering: Can we have a freakin' meeting where the attention is on us, not the men in our lives?

The setting couldn't be more perfect. At Tamar's house, the last hundred years clash stunningly. A faded, green Victorian couch is next to a midnight-blue recliner from the seventies, in pleather. The white plates our bagels sit upon are contemporary squares, though our coffee is poured into mismatched cups and saucers from the thirties. We drink mimosas out of mugs that say things like: *Did You Get Your Flu Shot?* (Tamar works in health policy.) The fizzy booze helps female desire bubble up. Safe topics first: We want dresses with pockets, a decent croissant, less expensive childcare, toastier temperatures in conference ballrooms, and partners who take our birthdays seriously. I feel like we're at a consciousness-raising group, updated. Women just rapping about our lives.

But now it's time to talk about bonking.

Ama starts us off. She's a young woman from Ghana, Tamar's friend, whose delicate bones give her a regal expression. Her British accent helps the royalty effect. Ama has no need for anonymity. "Sorry, I realize you said to pick someone else's card, but is it all right if I ask what I want?"

"Sure," replies Tamar waving her long arms to reassure. She could be Angelica Huston's sister. "We don't even need the cards."

Don't we? Tamar is grinning at Ama. The *room* is grinning, so I decide to go with the flow.

Then Ama asks, "How do you keep the spark alive in a marriage?"

She goes on, "I'm getting married in six months, and I really want to know the secret. Is there a secret?" She surveys the room with long eyelashes that might be fake, but this woman is for real. She mostly directs her gaze at those of us over forty. We—the hags with husbands—are supposed to save her marriage. But us older chicks only eyeball each other, like we're passing a ball no one has the strength to throw. Finally, Patrise, a visual artist in chunky plastic jewelry, states carefully, "I think a lot of people slow down with attraction to a partner. It changes over time. You just . . ."

"You stop doing it," inserts Gina with perfect comic timing. A sixty-five-year-old yogini with long, gray hair and electric-blue boots, she's the oldest here. I watch her take a sip of her mimosa. She's still smiling from her levity, but her chest goes on a sad journey, all the way up and all the way down. I want to hug her.

"So you've all stopped shagging?" Ama asks, accusingly.

"Almost," Gina responds with a puckered mouth that looks like she's sipping a dry martini rather than orange juice and champagne.

"It gets complicated," I offer.

"It gets complicated by other things—like anger," says Gina, laughing uproariously as the wrinkled among us join in. It's not funny.

As the mirth dies down, I ponder which camp I'm in. I may be close to Gina's age, but I'm also a newlywed. Is it possible to hold onto the promise Ama will feel on her wedding day? Or am I just being naïve?

If that's the case, so be it. Following Ama's courage, I pick my own card out of the wicker basket and watch the card stock tremble. "Does anyone else have painful intercourse?" I ask, looking around as Ama had done. Then I ramble. It goes something like this: "What's going on is definitely related to childhood sexual abuse. Does anyone else experience, you know, pain?"

Silence follows. Nine women gawk at me, endlessly. Then Gina puts her mug down as a hand comes up, resting on her cheek. "Laura, I'm not sure if you're aware, but as women age, the tissues can become dry and thin. Past a certain age, pain is pretty common."

"I know," I say nodding, but her comment is like cold air on the back of my neck. "What I have is different," I say, explaining to Gina and the room that I've had these snags since forever, so I'm sure it's not an age thing. Also, I tell them all about my vaginismus. "Have any of you heard of vaginismus?" No one here has heard of it. I shut up after that because I'm trying to figure out why I'm annoyed. It's like Gina wants to throw my problems into a box. My whole life, I've felt my sexual response was supposed to fit into categories I didn't relate to. Maybe there *is* no category for me.

But am I certain? My friend's comment is not without merit. I'm forty-eight! Shouldn't I be getting my hormones checked, or whatever a person does when her period is regular but she's middle-aged? I'm just about to request more information from this group when Teresa, a woman with round coal eyes, who said she was forty-three and born in Guatemala when we introduced ourselves, but has said nothing since, dives into a monologue. It's barely loud enough to hear, even though I'm right next to her. "You asked about painful sex. For me, making love is painful. I was also sexually abused—when I was really little. Tim, that's my husband, he's been dealing with this since we got together. But it's awful. And I feel bad. But what can I do? It's awful, all the time. It doesn't matter what I do. I mean, he's patient. He really is. I don't fault him for losing patience. It's just awful."

After her confession, she stares at each of us, and we stare back. Everyone is a little shocked, I think. Then Teresa's eyes go down.

"Thank you," I whisper to her, patting her arm, which feels cold. She doesn't look up. In fact, the crowd has now mirrored her introspective posture—chins down with focus on interior things, probably our own raw, unintelligible scenes.

When Tamar and I concocted the brunch at our tea date, she donned her health policy hat, rattling off statistics: one in four women have been sexually abused before the age of eighteen, one in six have been raped, one-third of assault survivors contemplate suicide, two-thirds experience chronic emotional distress. Contemplating these stats now, I'm not sure our bedroom experiences are part of these data. Do we have language and numbers that speak to our bodies in the aftermath? I thought I was breaking this cycle by speaking up about my own struggles, but my eyes are on the floor too.

Gratefully, the next inquiry breaks the mood.

It doesn't come to us immediately, though. First, there's low-volume eating and drinking. But ultimately, Cara puts her hand in the wicker basket and actually pulls out another's card. Yay for protocol. And yay for Cara, a millennial with long, red hair and a bright, dimpled face. "I love this," she says right after reading the question to herself. Then she goes for it: "What is a healthy sex life?"

"So let's talk about health," she adds, snapping her fingers like she's at a jazz club that even predates her parents.

Her gesture makes giggles reemerge. I reach for a brownie and notice others going in for their own sugar fix. Amidst the revelry, Cara, whose eyes are still infectiously lit up, tosses out a punch line, "My husband thinks a healthy sex life is at least once a day." She leans back on the Victorian couch, enjoying the guffaws she set off.

Slowly, Gina narrows her eyes and mouth toward Cara. "Is he making you sleep with him *every day*?"

"No! Of course not!" Cara replies, crossing her arms. "I just feel bad. Obviously, he's, you know, turned on."

"How often do *you* want to have sex?" asks Patrise, the painter. She's been married many years.

"I'm not sure," Cara says flicking her eyes around the room. Perhaps she's hoping we have an exact figure for her.

I suppose we do, in a way. Rapid-fire advice ricochets off the mismatched furniture. However, the message is singular—what Cara's husband is requesting is unreasonable. Cara listens and nods, but it seems she might cry.

Gina, meanwhile, starts clenching her fists, "I'm so mad about inequity, you know? Why do men have the right to be more powerful?"

"Because they are weak!" says Teresa, no longer looking down.

"They're afraid," chimes in Patrise.

"It's the patriarchy!" The room echoes with multiple shouts, as complaints pile up: *Why do they honk at us in the street? How come they leer at our nipples? Why do they violate so many of us?*

I let myself get carried by this current, though I'm cringing at the same time. Too often, I'm uncomfortable with mass displays of female rage, like here, where I hover above the increasingly red faces, feeling it's wrong to be aloof but unable to stop myself. I start thinking of Marion, a therapist I saw in the nineties. Marion wanted me to express my anger, which she thought was repressed. Hands on hips, peering at me through the frame of her farm-blond hair, she would thrust her pelvis at me, asking me to imitate her. "Fuck you," she'd say. "Fuck you. Fuck you. Fuck you." When I told her I felt only pity for the pervs who abused me—when I said I no longer hated the male gender after my celibacy year—she didn't believe me.

Maybe she was right. All of a sudden my floating body joins the mass of joined females below because not being furious at men seems bonkers.

"FUCK YOU, PATRIARCHY," I shout into the still-pissed-off cacophony. But what I'm really saying is: *Fuck you, Cara's horny husband. Fuck you, Dad. And fuck you, Kurt, for thinking you could stick your dick in some random woman simply because she was available. Fuck you for thinking you could get away with that shit.*

My organs feel healthy, like blood can travel freely through them. I feel like a car-flipping superhero. But then I recall another aspect of my time with Marion. She wasn't just interested in general rage. She wanted me to access what I'd felt as a child when I conjured violent fantasies. They were always the same. I was nineteen-years-old with hot-pink nails. I was using my fingernails to gouge out the eyes of Tammy's grandfather.

This memory halts my vital functions. Like my liver has been unplugged. Of course, those harming feelings exist within me. I know exactly where they live too—in my crotch, which is perpetually fighting back. My vagina isn't just frightened, she's seething.

But what to do about it?

The shitty behavior of men dominates our dialogue until the end of our Brunch. And I'm pretty sure it'll continue through all my living days.

Once Tamar and I are alone cleaning up, she offers more statistics, visibly still revved from the frenzy. Her Angelica Houston arms wave around a mouth that's twisted. She says it's important to not just be a feminist but to be an activist. I agree! But what does *my* activism look like? I refuse to be trapped by a need to make men bleed.

Still drying dishes, a solution comes to me, more possibility than conclusion: Whatever resentment I have toward Kurt, and Father, and patriarchy, why can't I roll it into a goal? Why can't I fight my own way?

Turn:

Fuck You

Into:

Fuck Me—The Way I Like

I love this transformation.

I have three more months to make it happen.

Outside Tamar's building, the cold air puts my progress in perspective.

Yikes!

Only three months.

Tips for *Your* Pleasure Plan

Something to Try:

Two main reasons people don't talk to their friends about intimacy issues are shame and fear of betraying a partner. If either of these are coming up for you, try confiding in just one friend. Afterward, journal about how you felt.

Journal Prompts:

1. Are you comfortable talking to your friends about what's going on in your sex life?

   _____

   _____

   _____

2. If you're not comfortable, is there anyone you might approach for guidance, especially someone who is nonjudgmental and has some knowledge of these areas?

   _____

   _____

   _____

3. What questions would you ask this person about sex?

   _____

   _____

   _____

4. Might menopause, perimenopause, or other hormonal changes be part of what's going on? (If so, see the Appendix for more about this.)

   _____

   _____

   _____

8

The Couples Retreat

"So what's the take-away?"

That's what Ari wants to know. Ari is the Artistic Director of the theater that's commissioned my play. He's Shirley's amazing boss. The three of us are crammed into his office, stuffed between shelves of scripts, where I've just presented for them the first draft of my sexual healing play. I've named it *Married Sex*. Reading this piece aloud was a blast. Even with limited space, I stood in front of the closed door, acting out each character: the hypnotist, the gynecologist, the Sex Brunch maidens.

But now, scrutinizing the story with my colleagues, it's clear my dramatic creation is only a series of scraps, not a cohesive narrative. These wise theater folk urge me to find a conclusive ending, one in which I'm resurrected by overcoming trauma. I assure them I'm looking for the very same thing.

On my way out, Ari says, "By the way, has Kurt seen this?"

A twinge of panic runs up my spine. I explain that he's seen the opening, but I didn't provide more pages because the quest didn't add up yet. I was waiting for the concrete result that he, Shirley, and I were just discussing. My logic vis-à-vis my husband seemed sound but Ari's comment has me worried. I ask my collaborators, "Do you think the play is problematic?"

"No, not at all," says Shirley, glancing at her colleague and then me. "It's just pretty personal. That's all."

I promise them when it comes together, I'll show my mate. Then I wander onto the street, anxious about how I'm going to mend soul, psyche, and vajayjay in the limited time I have left. Once this drama project is over, so is my recovery. Without deadlines and accountability—without the pressure to take risks—I don't see myself advancing. This is my only method of ever moving forward.

Could this method be enough?

Walking home, I want to believe my strategy has a chance of working, as long as I follow the map I've created—my list of experts. *Stop overthinking this*, I think, overly. I bring to mind the next listed modality, which might fix me by knitting together my plethora of strands.

This damn plethora of strands.

I just have to convince Kurt to try another wild tantric adventure.

My persuasive shot arrives that Sunday while my husband and I stroll to our neighborhood farmer's market. Now that Kurt has confessed his indiscretion, he's warmed to my project. He even stopped calling it "pathological," though this word has become a house meme. *Let's brown the chicken more; right now it's pathological. Can you get me a fresh towel? This one's pathological.* Today, on our jaunt, my guy seems extra attentive by not plowing ahead, a bad habit of his. He's with me, hip to hip. The moment couldn't be better to suggest a scary erotic experience.

"Schmookie?" I float. *Schmookie* is a recent addition to our endearments.

"Yes, Schmookie."

"Schmookie, I'm not sure if you'd be into this, but I found a retreat in Florida that helps couples with intimacy. In fact, it's called the *Intimacy Retreat*."

"Okay…"

"The thing is, it mildly involves tantra, and we'd have to use savings, but I have some money I can use from the theater." As I continue, I highlight the benign—no nudity, no public nooky, a man as co-facilitator. I stress the stupendous—useful tips for being close, and we would get to see Scott. Scott is Kurt's best friend who, after being diagnosed with cancer a few months ago, is convalescing in the Sunshine State, near the workshop site.

Another bonus I mention is that we'd escape the November chill.

"When is it?" asks Kurt, as he inspects fruits and veggies already shrunken due to the cold.

"Thank you," I squeal prematurely, squeezing him around the waist.

"Not the kidneys!" he cautions, reminding me that guys too can be delicate.

Then we work out the logistics for our trip. And just like that, we have a bit of a plan, together.

Three weeks later we arrive in paradise, which is what this private beach community evokes with its waving palm trees; sea-soaked air; salmon and aquamarine homes; and pristine white sand. We check into a stucco bungalow, steps from the water. I already feel restored.

That evening, Diana, who is co-facilitating, welcomes us into her home with laughter. I like her. She's less mystical than Francesca. I can imagine running into her at a supermarket on a Tuesday, this gorgeous woman who makes nothing of it—in her loose-fitting white pants, long-sleeve black top, untamed curls, and only a touch of makeup. I hope there will be time to work with her solo.

Richard, her husband, comes up behind, placing his hands on her shoulders. Tall, tan, and balding, he's also low-key but full of light. His white linen shirt and beige khakis blend with his wife's ensemble. They are a team. Together, this duo assembles us—six couples total—into a circle in their living room. I smile at the group, and also the meditation cushion I'm sitting on, the Oriental rugs scattered throughout, the remarkable sunset visible from an adjoining glassed-in porch. Kurt is happy too. He clasps my hand because he thinks we made the right choice. Diana rings a gong to begin.

Introductions are first, and out comes my *Pleasure Plan* journal—to record what people say. I know, it's creepy, but I've never sat with conjugal partners disclosing like this before. Two forty-something scientists from Ohio, both in too-large glasses, have never had a sensual spark. A Baptist minister and his wife, seventy-plus, rarely make love because, as the wife declares, "I'm a grandmother." A pair of Grateful Dead fans, who still excitedly follow the band, find their romance at a standstill. Another couple suffers from depression, mutually. And then there are the Austrians. These lovers, close to sixty and decked out in lululemon, are "absolutely crazy" about acquiring new techniques. When it's my turn to speak, inspired by the Austrians' attitude, I stress my desire to learn, ending with, "I'm thankful my *beloved* Kurt is here with me." I got this B-word from Diana. It's a very good word.

Diana has lots of intriguing language—and ideas. Seated on her own meditation cushion, she informs us that during the weekend, we will bond with our beloved in three intersecting ways, represented by three blazing candles in front of her and Richard: red for *Sex*, green for *Heart*, and purple for *Spirit*. "It's common for couples to connect in one of these areas, or even two. But not all three," she says.

Everyone nods.

I love those flames. I imagine them being the integration I'm searching for. Our homework tonight sets the stage. In the privacy of our chosen lodging, we are to stand before each other without clothes, saying "Sex, Heart, Spirit," while touching corresponding places on the body—genitals for *Sex*, chest for *Heart*, and between the eyes for *Spirit*.

At our cottage, a little later, Kurt and I get right to it. Disrobing fast, we leave the overhead light on to take each other in. Lamps add a needed cozy glow to the fish motif on the pale-green bedspread, the kitschy-charm paintings of sandy tableau.

"Sex, Heart, Spirit," I say into Kurt's eyes, where I climb into a midnight blue universe of guilt, and love, and insecurity, and mirth, and goodness, and fear of losing me.

"Sex, Heart, Spirit," he repeats.

As we continue intoning, as he beholds me as well, I don't know what he deciphers in my own universe. I hope he sees I'm thrilled to be naked with him via every avenue we discover here.

We fall asleep curled around each other.

The next morning, while meandering on the beach with Kurt before the workshop, I begin revealing what I have so far in my play, asking him for help: How should the cure coalesce? "On the beach with the couple swimming," he suggests. In other words, a setting similar to here, the shoreline behind our bungalow. I adore this poetry but have no idea how to get there, non-poetically. A kiss confirms it, nonetheless. Leaving the sea for an instructive living room, we are hand in hand.

When we get to the retreat house, however, we're met with segregation. The males are ushered to another room while we females are told to pick out a scarf we'll adorn later. These exercises are how we'll connect to our lovers through *Heart*.

Shortly after, our men return, each carrying a square plastic basin, overflowing with water. Richard oversees the placement of these objects on the floor. Gals are to pull up a chair next to our guy's little bath as Richard drops lavender oil into each tub, where rose petals float on the surface. Once the females are seated, our facilitator requests that we submerge our feet because "Women love to be pampered."

"Not all women," challenges the minister whose wife, the night before, described herself as *a grandmother*. "I keep telling her she deserves pleasure," he announces to the room with his arms lifted toward the heavens, like he's hoping God and the folks around him will talk sense into her. His spouse seems embarrassed, pursing her lips in the harsh sun streaming in from the porch. I feel bad for her, especially not being able to receive delight.

But focusing a few minutes later on my own mini-sea, my toes wiggling in water, I'm just as tense—in spite of the delicious temperature, Kurt's capable hands, and a Provençal field drifting up to my face from the oil. In lieu of surrendering, I wonder what percentage of women struggle with pleasure, of all kinds. Frankly, it's a miracle any of us prioritize feeling good. Matriarchs, for generations, were not allowed to enjoy being alive.

My own mom wouldn't even order a meal in a restaurant. She claimed she wasn't hungry, but then she'd devour three french fries someone had left on his plate. Occasionally, she *would* ask for individual food, which she'd savor—"Mmm, mmm, mmm"—before spitting it into her hand after chewing, so she wouldn't "get fat." Patting her soft round belly, she'd emphasize how weight never came off, and that's why she opted for polyester pantsuits with elasticized waists. She purchased these (often-stained) items at thrift shops. For me, it was silk shorts from Saks Fifth Avenue, and all those ballet lessons, plus instruction in jazz, tap, singing, and acting. I grew up indulged—and guilty. This insight is not new. But another realization starts burrowing, slowly, into my stomach, making me feel like I ate too much. Is my pelvic pain self-inflicted? Am I punishing myself for taking too much as a child?

When the footbath ends, I'm relieved. It's a great experience. I just don't know how to savor it. The next activity appears easier, when it comes to *Heart*. We're going to enchant the men.

Once the guys leave (to empty their basins), Diana, touching the turquoise beads around her neck, tells us it's time for us ladies to adorn ourselves with the fabrics we chose earlier. We're to dance for our male partners. A sparkly shawl I've already claimed is restless on a chair. The color of blueberries, it has reflective pieces, like minuscule mirrors embedded throughout. I know Kurt will appreciate the intricate design because men are so visual.

The second our spouses reenter, Arabic music with visceral drums permeates the room. My love materializes, and we embrace. Then I break away to sway for him and turn around so he can study my ass, which hikes up from side to side. Since my year of celibacy—when I made peace with the male gaze—I've retained a strange comfort with objectification. To me, it's a victory: I've won the right to be appreciated without feeling victimized. Is this internalized oppression? Possibly. But I find that categorization simplistic. Arousal, as little as I understand it, often involves a body display—in sum but also in parts. Excitement for all involved. Or that's how it is for me. Accordingly, I run my hands through my hair, and tickle it down each arm, keeping my focus on Kurt, who is also swaying rhythmically. He looks good today, in his polo shirt and cargo shorts.

I start wondering what other men are wearing. Their attire didn't register when I saw them earlier. It didn't seem significant, but now it does. I could look, no? Why can't I look?

An embarrassed grin takes over my head, as I peer at other men. Diana said not to, but my sneak-peek is subtle. It's enough to see so much. Shoulders flow into biceps that surge into powerful wrists. Hips free up and the sinew of thighs presses into pants and shorts.

"Don't go for passion."

When my mother warned me, using this phrase, I interpreted it to mean: *Turn off your senses. Do it to stay with men with whom you have no chemistry.* Mom's advice reverberated what I found in bestselling books, in romance movies, in TV sitcoms, in stuffy psychology seminars, and during chatter in stinky-beer bars. Always the same idea: men are whipped up through their eyes but women are interested in emotions.

This concept still echoes around the zeitgeist.

Yet, on Diana and Richard's sun-porch dance floor, I think: *What if I'm also visual?* The entire cavity of my torso suddenly aches with desire, and grief. Would I have gone so long without love if I'd allowed myself a full spectrum of vibrancy?

Furtively boogying with six guys, my own included, music faster now, I let my body spread wide for a million points of visual stimuli.

I'm ravenous for the globe, pulled in through taste, touch, sound, and smell. Sweat saturates my temples and pits by the time the music fades down. I place my hands in prayer position and bow—to Kurt, our facilitators, and to *Heart*. The heart of who I possibly am as an erotic person.

I know it's just the beginning, but what just happened seems the center of some knowing.

And guess what?

It's time for *Sex*.

Back in the circle our facilitators talk about the importance of carnal connection to our mate. Nice! My body still feels porous and vital. An amber glow—emanating from my brain—infuses the room. But then I discover the specifics of what we're about to do. We'll be massaging the yoni (female genitalia) and lingam (male genitalia). First, the yoni, which we'll learn about through demo, followed by a partner practice in our hotel rooms.

Even before the demonstration begins, my groin clenches in dread. I despise fingers inside me; they hurt even more than dicks. But what if the forthcoming exercise will not be "fingering," but a flowering based on the heart expansion I just experienced? I try to keep an open mind and pelvic floor.

Perhaps it'll be fine if we follow along with the paper. Our workshop leaders presently pass out a diagram depicting a woman's sex organs, like you are peering down onto this region. Then, with Diana reclining on a yoga mat and throw pillows, with Richard kneeling beside, they get more nitty-gritty. Thankfully, Diana's loose cotton pants stay on as she and Richard point out a woman's anatomy: outer and inner labia, clitoral button and hood, internal clitoris, urethra, vaginal opening, G-spot, and anus.

I try to recall if I've ever had sex education like this. It certainly wasn't in seventh grade, when our Health teacher told us about menses and intercourse, but mostly talked about coming home from war with shrapnel in his leg and "shell shock" in his soul.

That same summer, starved for sensual know-how, I begged my friends to let me play Truth or Dare with them, even though they said I was too flat-chested and shy. Finally, they relented. For weeks, lit by moonlight and cigarette butts, we'd sit on the beach imparting Dares (we never messed with Truth). A classic Dare was this: *Swim forty feet into the ocean or make out with Tommy behind the sand dune.* We always chose the tongue fest. One day, Tommy, the boy with Marlboro breath I liked best, said I didn't know how to kiss. When I asked him to elaborate, he said. "You should kiss like Lisa." I was too mortified to ask Lisa for advice.

I should have asked. At fourteen, Lisa probably had more knowledge than I have right now at Diana and Richard's. I'm sure of it as I try retaining the female bits our hosts are meticulously detailing. I wish I could study pussy for a week. Before I know it, Kurt and I are retiring to our rooms for the private portion of this activity.

Once we lock the door, bright red silky panties sneak their way to my body. I purchased these for ten dollars on Amazon, an effort to grow my trousseau, economically. I recline in my cute cover-up until Kurt remarks we can't do the assignment this way.

"Oh yeah, right," I say innocently, pretending I'm not fending off attack. Then I take my undies off slowly, opening my knees in a butterfly pose as they showed us. My legs are fidgety like at the gynecologist. Also, my vulva feels cold because I'm frigid in every possible way. It doesn't help that Kurt is consulting the handout.

"You don't need no stupid paper," I tease as if I'm a normal woman. "You *know* what's there. Don't you?"

"I thought I did," he says, studying the picture upside down, a Kurt joke I now understand.

"You'll be fine!" I reassure him, patting the bed, though I'm the person who needs reassuring. The towel we've placed on the comforter is next to a bottle of lube we brought from home.

"You ready? Here I come." Kurt pretends to dive onto the bed.

Before we left for our private dwelling, Richard had told us: "Make sure you don't just stick your hand in there. You need to spend a lot of time caressing the whole body. Then, slowly, work your way toward touching the vulva. Spend lots of time massaging externally before you begin entering."

I want to get this over with quickly, however, so I have my partner penetrate me without a lot of fanfare. As he inserts one finger, I focus on my senses because my face is wincing. Taste…smell…sight… sound…the room pleases me aesthetically, but there's an intruder pillaging every artifact depicted in the drawing. All I feel is burning like my sacred chamber is aflame. Arson in the temple.

I put up with it for five minutes, until I pull out his paw.

"That's it?" he asks.

"Yup." My silk is back on instantly. Best ten dollars ever. "I think I'm going to nap," I say. Facing away from resting Kurt, I attempt a slumber escape from what just ensued. But, of course, I can't sleep. All my brain is interested in is a conversation from last week. The call nobody knows about.

I had phoned a sex therapist, another scary practitioner on *The Pleasure Plan* list. A rash on my elbow appeared as I dialed and pondered: *Did these professionals sleep with their clients?* I really didn't know.

Still, I managed to leave a message. When the sexpert called me back, I happened to be at a Panera. I had no intention of having sex therapy amidst melting paninis, plus a nearby booth where college kids were studying Spanish. But Dr. Goldberg began grilling me. Clearing my mouth of cheese, whispering, I told her about painful intercourse.

"Okay, stop," she said immediately. "You have pelvic pain?"

"Yeah."

"I don't treat anyone with pelvic pain."

The rash suddenly returned on my elbow, contagiously, like I could infect that table of language students. Dr. Goldberg told me I should try physical therapy, which I didn't understand. All I comprehended was this: I was too broken for even a sex therapist.

Recalling this encounter in Florida, still balled up on the mint comforter, I start rousing myself for the next part of the workshop. We're to report on our vaginas.

An hour later, convened in Diana's and Richard's early dusk living room, this is what I hear: "Amazing undulations." "I felt cherished." "Very, very nice." When my turn arrives, I awkwardly confess my troubles. Diana fixes her liquid eyes on me, saying, "Unfortunately, I'm not an expert on painful sex." She adds she would like to offer me resources. But, at that moment, I'm too overwhelmed—by my damaged yoni, the pressure I've put on myself to heal in only six months, and the remaining *Pleasure Plan* professionals I still haven't gotten to.

That's why it doesn't make sense what I'm hoping for after dinner. Lingering in Diana and Richard's kitchen, after the yummy meal they just served us, I wait for the Austrian babe, the Grateful Dead mama, and Grandma to come over with kind words or advice. None do.

As Kurt and I walk back to our room, silently, I have to conclude that when it comes to a *Sex* communion, I am still very much a freak.

So what about tomorrow?

Tomorrow, our final day, we will explore *Spirit*. Will I be able to move past my dysfunction in order to connect?

❋

Entering the house the next morning, we find it's been transformed —no more meditation seats. As we stand around sipping coffee, Richard informs us we're going to learn how to make love every day. Spiky adrenaline surges through me. *Isn't limited humping bad enough? Once a week, or every couple of weeks.* Our host continues, speaking about tantra. Communing with our mates—via *Sex*, *Heart*, and *Spirit*—is the essence of tantra.

In truth, both he and Diana have been saying this since we arrived, but my head is only just starting to assemble their vast knowledge and know-how, which is terrific because that's what I came here for—to finally fit pieces together.

Our teachers lead us then to their back porch, which has also been modified. In place of mid-century modern furniture, there are now six massage tables. Against the sliding glass door is a banquet crowded with delectable items: sliced fruit, faux fur, a jar of Hershey's chocolate sauce, essential oils, bells, and more. Describing what to do with these, Diana says, "Don't wait until your lover is dying to give this personal attention." I take this to mean our partners are facets of the Divine who are given to us for a short time. By honoring their bodies, we honor their souls.

I'm the first soul on the table. As I recline, faceup, Kurt puts a satin blindfold on me, which makes me feel vulnerable. I fool around with inhalations and exhalations to calm my nerves. Then tout de suite, Kurt brings by some treats. Tiny bells are dangling close to my ears as a slice of cantaloupe enters my lips. It's followed by mango, which melts on my tongue. A scrap of fur traces and tickles my palm. As this stimulation continues, I melt a little too. But it's not just pleasure softening me. It's surprise. Every experience is intensified by the unexpected. It brings to mind a book I recently devoured, *Mating in Captivity* by Esther Perel. In this brilliant tome, the author says that Eros thrives in an atmosphere of novelty, as well as mystery, uncertainty, and even danger.

With Kurt feeding me more sensations. I begin pondering my cravings beyond more fruit, different fruit. I silently whisper to myself: *What am I jonesing for in bed?* My heart instantly beats forcefully, like I'm punching myself on the inside for daring to ask. I keep repeating my question, regardless, until a dormant little hunger awakens between my legs. More twinge than appetite, I follow its small rush of blood. After thirty years of screwing, I honestly do not know what I want. I float some possibilities: *Varied partners? BDSM? Rubber masks?*

Suddenly, I announce, "I'm done." It's not the masks that scare me, or maybe it is. "We can stop," I say getting off the table, even though my turn has not technically ended. *Do I really need to know what I desire?* God-honest arousal, my out-of-control heart is sure of it, would threaten my marriage.

I'm glad when we switch places, and Kurt hops on the table. As usual, I prefer this role. I march to the goodies, to let chocolate sauce fly. Boy, do I adore pouring Hershey's onto my hubby's thumb and licking it off. However, every time I go back to the yummy items, I have the same thought: *How long did it take to cut up all that cantaloupe?*

I pride myself on pleasing my guy, but I start wondering if I'm also lazy, only willing to go so far. In other words, receiving *and* giving are probably complicated for me.

I can see a path forward, however. *Just do the exercises.* If I replicate what they're teaching us this weekend—the exercises—might I improve sensual skills despite trauma and finicky genitalia? Maybe that's the case.

Just do the exercises.

"This is how you make love every day," Richard says at the end of the retreat. "Through footbaths, and dancing, and massages, through dedicated attention focused on our mates. By giving all of ourselves: *Sex, Heart,* and *Spirit.*"

Before Diana blows out the candles, she states again, "Don't wait until your beloved is dying before you give all of yourself."

Diana's and Richard's words ring through our rental car, as my husband and I drive through Florida to see our friend Scott, who, in recent weeks, has deteriorated considerably. His spouse, Vincent, put Scott in a nursing home.

After entering this facility, we see the couple in the clean, paneled dining hall. Scott is unrecognizable. He must have lost thirty pounds. With a gaunt visage and veiny arms, he speaks to us, beaming, but we can't grasp what he's saying. Words are clear but the string of them is nonsensical.

He is exquisitely taken care of. Vincent, who comes by daily, attends to Scott as we sit, trying to decode our buddy's non sequiturs. Vincent massages lotion on his partner's face and hands; he makes sure the fleece blanket stays up to his chin; he spoon-feeds Scott every morsel.

It's undeniable. Kurt and I will end up in a place like this too. In fact, such an arrangement is the definition of an excellent union—the privilege of helping someone die. Being lustful is very far away at this moment. But that's okay. As I just grasped at the retreat, this too is making love.

Once we exit the nursing home, Kurt and I meander, saying little. Sadness shortens my gaze and reels in all my tethers. I want to shut out this humid neighborhood, but Florida is a very horny state. It's hard not to notice the southern palm trees flirting like their cousins up north. The same with plants showing off their tropical decadence—salmon and eggplant, saffron mixed with busting-out yellow. And all the birds that left DC for the cold? They're down here whooping it up.

Unexpectedly, my nipples harden.

I wonder if this is similar to what I experienced while running in the park a few months back, talking dirty to myself on my iPhone. I realized then I was part of an erotic universe, where libidinous expressions abound. But libido is not just a survival instinct, as Freud would have it. It's a larger yearning for intimacy with an animating force keeping us going until it takes up residence elsewhere. Scott will become part of this all-abiding energy soon. I squeeze Kurt's hand.

I am not dying in a nursing home. Neither is my lover.

Not yet.

The *Heart* and *Spirit* connection I found this weekend is perfect, but it's not enough. I also want *Sex*—ravishing bonking; ecstatic emergence; exploding rockets beyond earth; big orgasms that annoy my neighbors. I want it all.

What will it take to finally have it all?

Tips for *Your* Pleasure Plan

Something to Try:

Set these out on a table: fruit, fabric, oils … or anything else that thrills the senses. You can be alone or with a partner.

The real trick here is making the effort and allotting enough time. Take your time and enjoy the exploration.

Journal Prompts:

1. If you expanded your concept of lovemaking—beyond the genitals—what would that look like?

   _____

   _____

   _____

2. What are all the ways you like to be sensually delighted?

   _____

   _____

   _____

3. Are you resistant to being generous with a lover? If so, why? Are you resistant to receiving pleasure from a lover? If so, why?

   _____

   _____

   _____

9

The Ocean

I'm sliding all over the highway on US 95, in an icy December rain. I'm about to do something crazy. I'm on my way to the garage where I was molested as a child, a spot in Brooklyn five hours from my home. It's time to vanquish my trauma by shocking it out of my body.

I've just reached the New Jersey Turnpike, almost halfway there. At the first rest stop, I pull off to order a fried chicken sandwich. I eat slowly, trying to re-conjure the logic that brought me to this point. It's the same reasoning that will keep me traveling North instead of South, back to where I came from.

It started at a military trauma conference, two weeks before. My army friend Pam invited me after I told her I thought I had PTSD. She was surprised. So was I when I first came up with it. During my decades of therapy, this diagnosis never came up. I think it's because I didn't exhibit common symptoms like flashbacks, nightmares, or hypervigilance on the street. I even double-checked if I had this disorder when I first embarked upon *The Pleasure Plan*, searching in the *Diagnostic and Statistical Manual*. Nope, I didn't meet the criteria. I did find my range of sexual dysfunctions, though, in a completely different section. There didn't seem to be a link. But after the couples retreat, and especially my failed yoni massage, I began suspecting I had another, unknown, traumatic stress disorder. I dubbed it *PTSD of the Vagina*. It was the only way I could explain my genitals to myself. Pam laughed at my diagnosis but arranged for me to attend this gathering, where the cutting edge of trauma recovery would be discussed.

My friend did not disappoint.

The morning of the conference, I sat in the darkened auditorium, taking in a very informative overview of where the trauma field stands at this moment, particularly from the perspective of the military, which does most of the PTSD research in the country. Experts emphasized two overlapping approaches they were most fond of—calming a patient's nervous system and helping this person process their trauma narrative.

That morning, we got to sample the former. Therapists, physicians, and other PTSD pros spoke about the sympathetic and parasympathetic nervous systems, two main branches of our autonomic nervous system. Activating the parasympathetic nervous system counteracts fight, flight, or freeze. It relaxes us. To that end, we did trauma-informed yoga, mindfulness meditation, and Emotional Freedom Technique (EFT). I was thrilled EFT was featured as I'd included it as part of *The Pleasure Plan* after hearing about its benefits for years. In EFT, you conjure an upsetting memory, or event, keeping it in your mind while you tap on nine points distributed throughout the body. In the dim, state-of-the-art auditorium, I conjured an unsettling argument with a friend. Then I tapped as instructed. Remarkably, after this exercise, I felt less upset.

After lunch, we ventured into the other half of healing, that is, how to process memories. That's when an extremely tall, white-haired psychiatrist took the stage. His favorite modality was a technique I'd never heard of—Prolonged Exposure, or PE. In Prolonged Exposure, a patient with traumatic stress is brought repeatedly back to the site of his or her trauma—usually through imagination or virtual reality—until this locale no longer controls a client's life.

I can do that myself, I thought, so excited I wanted to run through the halls of this corporate conference center. *An outing to my own personal traumaland.* Was I aware that a single visit did not qualify as PE? Sure. How could one exposure be considered *prolonged*? Real Prolonged Exposure would involve a therapist as well as months, or years, of treatment. I didn't want the actual experience. Or maybe I was just being DIY like my mom and the suction she applied to the family's nostrils. I didn't care. I had an instinct this experience would transform me. Wasn't this worth a shot? Yes!

"Yes!" is what got me on the road this morning.

"Yes!" has led me to this fried chicken sandwich at the rest stop—for protein, I tell myself. "Yes!" makes me stand in a stupidly long Starbuck's line so I can get more caffeinated. "Yes!" takes me over the slick, harrowing Verrazano Bridge. When I first got my driver's license at seventeen, making a successful solo trip over this grated connector meant I was safe to go anywhere.

And "Yes!" takes me off the highway, finally, in a very hard rain. I cruise past a commercial district, a slew of towering apartment buildings, my junior high school, and a playground. A wide, saturated road takes me to my old neighborhood. I pull onto my block at 4:30 on that Thursday afternoon.

In the remaining gray, slanted light, I see the familiar rows of brick houses, painted yellow, white, or red. The maple tree next to where I park my car, three doors from the horror house, is bare as I would expect this time of year. But it seems ominous, emerging from a pile of dark slush, remnants of a recent snowstorm.

I stay in my old Saab, a car Kurt got a good deal on last year (he wanted me to have a safe vehicle for my frequent trips to schools). I'd never had heated seats before. As I soak up the electrons, I can't imagine better technology.

I should turn off my engine but I don't. I just stare at the garage I'm supposed to enter as well as my own house right in front of where I parked. The fenced-in patio is still there. My parents sold our home twenty years ago. It's nice to imagine how my bedroom appears now. But that's not what I came here for. I'm having trouble believing in what I came here for.

You know what gets me out of that vehicle? It's the play. On the way over, I decided this visit would make a dynamite scene in my drama. The idea helped keep me on the road—along with "Yes!" I wasn't doing this for me; I was doing it for art. That's how it is with me.

Eventually opening the car door, I feel freezing rain pelt my nose. The hat I pull on smells like wet wool. I grip my umbrella tightly as I walk. It's only 200 feet but I go so slowly it might be 200 years until I get there. Ice chunks have made their way to my pancreas—that's how cold I feel. I'm not sure I will ever thaw.

When I reach the brick two-family abode that, rumor has it, my abuser built with his own hands, I encounter a white door with a small triangular window. Squinting in, all I see is blackness. I dare myself to ring the bell. Three times. No one comes to the door.

Stepping backward so I can view the entirety of this red house, I can't forget what I know. There's an apartment upstairs, and the two floors don't intersect. A gaggle of related siblings used to live in this upstairs stomping ground. I hung out with them, in those rooms, for years, avoiding the downstairs garage. Making sure I was nowhere near this lower hell was the centerpiece of my childhood.

With my heart beating uncomfortably in my throat, I climb the stairs to the upper apartment, where I see an elderly Asian woman in a housedress gaping at me. She's behind the glass of her storm door, which she opens halfway. I've practically memorized my spiel: "Hi, my name is Laura...." Taking in her slight smile, I am grateful Kurt coached me the night before. Originally, I wanted to say I'd been molested in this house, but Mr. Ethics insisted I lie—just this once. As a finale to my monologue, I say, "I have such good memories playing here. Would you mind if I come inside?"

"No English," she says loudly, with a bye-bye wave of her hand. Then she closes the door in my face. I stand there watching the steam from my rapid respiration, which does not warm me.

When I get back in the car, I'm shivering uncontrollably. Emotional Freedom Technique floats around my skull, the tapping, but I can't recall where the points are. So I just tremble, hoping the electric seats I activate will toast my ass. I desperately want to leave this nightmare scene because I've done what I could do. *Isn't it enough that I got here?*

An unwanted idea batters my head, though, like the frigid chunks still coming down. If I wait an hour or two, hypothetical people who live downstairs will return. In that way, I might still get into the garage. I drown out this ambition by revving my engine and exiting this awful block. Yet all I do is drive around and around my childhood neighborhood. I keep thinking of the house I just left. Not only my abuser's but my own, three doors down.

It's that fenced-in patio. My mother had it built after I was born so that I couldn't wander away and get hurt. She bragged about the wrought-iron fence, also meant to keep me from harm. But on one particular day it didn't.

∗

I was playing with my Barbie dolls, along with other kids from my block. It must have been a weekend, or even a block party, because most of my neighbors were outside, having a festive time.

Instinct made me look up from brushing Barbie's hair. It was Tammy's grandfather perusing my house from afar. I think I was four, so the abuse was still going on then—as long as he could find me. Now he had found me.

In white workman's overalls, covered with black and blue and yellow paint, in dirty boots, he played the part of voyeur, twenty yards away. It seemed to me he was deciding whether or not to approach. Glacially, he began sauntering in the direction of my patio. I was frozen with disbelief and indignation: *He's really coming over here?*

Then, my body picked itself up, practically reaching the summer sky. I flew inside my house.

I must have taken off without an excuse, just adrenaline and legs. I must have appeared distressed because Johnny, a boy from my street, ran after me. He was a curly haired blond, huge for his age. He seemed like an adult or a teen. Though, if I do the math, he was only about ten at the time. I have no notion why he apprehended me in the front entryway of my own two-family house, why he grabbed my arm.

"Hey? What's going on?" he asked.

"Nothing. I'm going inside." I pulled to get away from his grip.

Johnny bent down so he was my height. "Not so fast. Did something happen back there?"

"No!" My heart was beating so fast I thought I might faint. What if Tammy's grandfather came into my hallway? At least in my house, I could lock the door. "Let me go," I screamed at Johnny.

"Not unless you tell me what's wrong." At this point, my mother came out with her hair in rollers.

"What's the matter?" Mom said loudly, alarmed.

"I don't like him," I whispered to both of them.

"Who?" my mother asked.

"Him," I answered, not quite audibly.

Bending down like Johnny, she said, "Can you tell me who you're talking about?"

Johnny, playing savior again, or bully, opened the door so we three could see the patio. That's when I saw Tammy's grandfather's thick, splattered hands resting on the fence; a foot was poised on the concrete base as if he were posing for Pedophile Mechanics.

Johnny was catching on. Sort of.

"Him?" He got up close to my abuser, pulling me into the big patio with him. Mom followed. Then he used the moniker all the kids preferred. I don't think any of us knew this man's actual name, "Tammy's grandfather?" asked Johnny, pointing.

The old guy seemed to enjoy the attention. He was leaning his big belly into the fence. Other children had gathered around to decode the mystery. Suddenly, Johnny came up with a theory: "Maybe she's scared because he looks like a clown." The kids loved this. "Yup. He looks like a clown!" Their laughter hurt my skin, and I didn't know if I would ever get my heart to stop this dangerous beating. The pervert stayed a while, chuckling. Then he merrily strolled away.

I took that as my cue to run and hide.

*

I've spent so many years hiding. Years I lived in this community, and decades after. What if I no longer have to run?

I return to my block, parking in exactly the same spot—in front of my childhood home, three residences down from the garage. Again, I make my way to the white door, and again there is blackness in the triangular window. Then, shockingly, a woman opens the door. Her glowing complexion and sleek black hair tell me she is around twenty. Her long skirt and the fact that her locks are a wig tell me she is one of the Orthodox Jews who have lived in this neighborhood since my childhood.

My monologue feels smoother now, but my inner being is jagged and gyrating.

"Come in," says the woman when my speech ends. "I don't mind."

And that's how I find myself back where I was repeatedly molested when I was four. I'm back in the garage—with one catch. There Is No Garage.

Upon entering, I can see the zone I was hunting for has been remodeled. A short entry vestibule opens into a living room. I stand in this second room, rotating 360 degrees. "Thank you so much for letting me look around," I say smiling at the young woman. Her house smells like chicken baking in the oven, with carrots.

"Is this how you remember it?" she asks.

"Yeah. Pretty much." I keep fake grinning but stop talking. Too many of my resources are trying to find the barrel. This black metal object contained paint. Around three feet tall and two feet in diameter, it's the pedestal where I stood. But first, the old man picked me up with calloused hands. He pulled down my pants. He pushed up my top. I've never buried this memory: the damp chill; the stench of paint and turpentine; the trapped girl staring at her exposed nipples and what her mother called a "pupi."

I do not locate the black barrel in this present home. But I *can* pinpoint where it once resided. On that exact spot is a small wooden desk with chrome legs.

I turn 180 degrees. Opposite the barrel in my psyche is the slimy concrete wall. That's where the pedophile leered at my body while taking out his penis. Against that same surface, now, is a white bookcase.

"It's such a lovely home," I tell the woman.

It's only a bookcase and a desk, I tell myself.

It's only a bookcase and a desk.

I can't stop staring at this everyman office. One thing is certain—this furniture was all bought at IKEA.

But what about the pre-IKEA items? The Garage. The Barrel. The Wall. I'm catching on: these objects have been transformed by the passage of time.

Have I?

After thanking the nice lady, I drive to the beach, just a few streets away. I want to see the water. It's still pouring as I get out of my car, but not icy like before. I open my umbrella, and wind from the sea knocks it inside out. Straightening this protection, I inhale the salty waves, which are crashing but not excessively. This is an aspect of living here I always loved—the ocean.

Ocean is how I always thought of this body of water, but it's not technically true. This section of the Atlantic coast is an inlet named Gravesend Bay. Gravesend Bay becomes the Hudson River, which becomes the Atlantic, which connects to all the fluid on our planet. None of us are just the size of ourselves.

As the minutes pass, I become soaked but I don't move because I can handle it. My umbrella has stopped functioning. It might completely collapse in the wind. But not me. I'm tall here, taller than I've ever been. I feel gangly like a teenager who's grown six inches in the past two hours. I'm as gargantuan as the lifeguard chair standing nearby. I used to sit on that perch, peering out over the sea and dreaming of life beyond this tiny, haunted place.

For a moment, I consider climbing up to its lofty height. I even know what I would think about when I got there: *being here means something.*

It means my bones are longer. It means there's ocean in my lungs. In that moment, I can't breathe. Or I've never taken such full breaths before.

I think this might be courage.

Tips for *Your* Pleasure Plan

Something to Try:

Write a story about your sexual healing as if it has already taken place—you're looking back on it. Put your story in the past tense. Include what you've learned! Read this to yourself, and note how you feel.

Journal Prompts:

1. Is there a story you're telling yourself about your erotic self?

   _____

   _____

   _____

2. Do you ever use your story to protect yourself?

   _____

   _____

   _____

3. If you wrote a new story, what would happen?

   _____

   _____

   _____

10

The Play

There's one more practitioner I want to see before I finish a final draft of my play—a trauma therapist. She's the last person on *The Pleasure Plan* list. I need her. My play needs her. After spreading my current text on the rug, printing paper stares back at me with single-spaced audacity. I try moving scenes around, hunting for that elusive, curative conclusion. But this hot, dramatic mess is still silly fragments. That's why I'm glad I have a piece left that might complete this healing puzzle.

I should have contacted Dr. Gregori at the beginning of my odyssey. In my many years of therapy, I never sat down with an expert on childhood sexual abuse. The closest I came was working recently with another type of trauma professional. In keeping with my commitment to all seven practitioners on my list, I had three sessions of EMDR in the last month. It was interesting. But the therapist, Dr. Valansky, wanted to focus on reprocessing my abuse story. I didn't feel I needed this, especially after my trip to Brooklyn.

I'm hoping Dr. Gregori is different.

The woman I encounter in her waiting room—with short, silver hair and long, tweed shirt—holds promise. She shakes my hand firmly.

There's nary a smile. Leading me to her inner chamber, I feel like I've been summoned to the principal's office. I find her low-pitched voice authoritative as well: "So tell me what brings you here."

I let it pour out of me, everything I can think of, while this serious pro takes notes. When my vessel is empty and weak, I sip from the bottle of water she gave me before I sat down. The scratch of her pen, the white walls, the glass side table strewn with *Psychology Today* magazines, they portend a seasoned analysis. Indeed, when Dr. Gregori looks up, she has a proclamation. "I don't think there's *anything* wrong with you. In fact, there never was."

"But what about my abuse?" I ask, incredulously. I offer again the highlights of the story I've just spent twenty minutes telling her—being molested by three men, on and on. When I get to the phrase haunting me for forty years—Mom saying, "That's what men are like; don't go near him"—Dr. Gregori's mouth turns up for the first time. Light shoots out of her black eyes: "She was right," the doctor says.

"She was right?"

"Yes!" The doctor nods vigorously, agreeing with my mother's abandonment. "You needed to know how to protect yourself." Her cheek-to-cheek smile conveys more friendliness than she's shown so far. Her teeth are almost white. "This is what survivors need more than anything else—agency. You learned agency."

Every ounce of me collapses into the gray couch. This therapist's spin on my history makes my past even heavier than it already is by adding this layer of perplexity. At the very least, I was certain how to contextualize what happened to me. Now, I'm unmoored, and it wears me down. I want to burrow into the textured fabric beneath me. But there's no time for rest. If I have no trauma, then how can I be treated? And if I can't be treated, how will I ever be repaired?

Perhaps she missed key details. I begin telling her about waters I rarely wade into—my mother scolding me, as a young child, for going around the house in my underwear. "Don't walk around with your pants off in front of your father." Yes, even my dad was capable of impropriety, even incest, according to my mother.

The doctor sticks with her assessment though and goes further. She's absolutely "thrilled" I'm writing a play about my odyssey. As for my current problems—that I still hate coupling, that I'm afraid of virility, that it's like I'm being raped every time I dabble in intercourse—she is not concerned. "You're doing everything right," she assures me.

Time to bring out the big guns. For the first time, I mention my self-diagnosis, PTSD of the Vagina. Dr. Gregori laughs even harder than my friend Pam, actually slapping a thigh. "Clever, but not how it works," she informs me. This expert insists I don't have *any* variety of post-traumatic stress disorder. "Just keep doing what you're doing," she concludes as I write out an exorbitant check.

The distance between that visit and my public presentation is less than a week. Typing at my desk the last day before I go live, beating this play into final form, I try maintaining Gregori's encouragement—her belief in my agency. It's hard not to notice what's spitting out of my printer, however. It does not resolve my loins.

Maybe it doesn't have to.

All of a sudden, an epiphany shoots down my vertebrae, concerning performance.

It wasn't just hands that harmed me; it was eyes.

Riffing on this, I ponder: Can eyeballs be used to reverse my psychological mutation? Possibly. A group of people witness how I vanquished an original gaze. This just might be what heals me. As I get ready for showtime, I prepare myself for breakthrough.

Performing Married Sex

A Play-Within-a-Play About a Play

Setting: A midsize theater in Washington, DC.

At Rise: Laura Zam, a solo performer, enters the stage in black pants, a black long-sleeve T-shirt, and a royal blue vest. Her hair is tied back, and she's wearing minimal makeup. It's a neutral countenance befitting someone who will transform. She addresses the audience directly.

LAURA

Guess what? I'm married!
After thirty years of disastrous romantic luck, someone that I love also loves me.

The performer throws her arms up in victory. She takes in her adoring fans, half of whom she doesn't know because they've come to see the play that will follow hers. Her strength is for the masses though, whoever they are. Spotlight on herself, the thespian continues her first monologue, syncing voice, body, mind, and artistic vision. It takes a tremendous amount of sweat to be a hundred percent herself, but theater inspires her to express everything she's mastered since her mother took her to the Little Theater School. The audience gets it. They get her. Except for one. A woman in the front row is sleeping. The front row! The actress redirects her energies; she's at her first physical transformation—her forte. She dons pretend glasses and throws her shoulders back so she can become her horny husband.

KURT

What do you say we stick it in?

The audience explodes in laughter, except the sleeping woman. The performer glares at this lady who can't see her, of course, because this rude spectator's eyes are closed. It doesn't matter. Even with sweat sticking to her spine, and pooling in her panties, Laura is human potential. Superhuman potential. She is a channel for the star-force of the universe. Nonetheless, a man stands and starts putting on his coat. The creatrix continues her lines as she watches this audience member make his way to the aisle so he can leave the theater. He's old, so his exit is a long shuffle with a winter coat draped over his arms.

I HAVE A RIGHT TO BE HERE, *she yells at the slow walker but only in her head because she has art to present. For the remainder of the play, the thespian transitions in and out of characters, including a hypnotist, a Tantrika, and a gynecologist. Twenty-one people in all. With spittle sprayed on her crowd, and perspiration dripping onto the stage, she transforms twenty-one different ways. More people fall asleep, throughout. Others are frowning with consternation and constipation.*

The last monologue has arrived. The performer despises the people watching her, but she gives this text what she has.

LAURA

Kurt and I end up on a beach. We swim together. We swim for our lives.

The lights slowly fade to black. In the darkness, Laura, the performer, pants from exhaustion. She notices that her panting is like other panting she's done. She is utterly unchanged.

End of Play

I need to find Kurt. I'm off the stage now, through the dressing room, and into the lobby. I don't even know what I want from him. Kind words? A hug? Definitely a hug. Also, dramaturgical analysis. He's great at that. I have *not* been healed by this project, it's true, but might this endeavor continue? I'm having trouble believing *The Pleasure Plan* is now over, that I no longer have this method of getting unstuck.

I don't see my husband anywhere. I do encounter strangers. None will meet my eyes. I feel like I've spent the last ninety minutes lifting up my skirt and exposing myself, pathologically.

Gamely, a few friends rush over to me. Gayle is here, along with Stacey and some other yoga buddies. A few women from the Sex Brunch showed up. Everyone's comments blend together:

"Wow."

"Good for you."

"That was sooo brave."

I don't understand where my husband is. And now I have to stop looking. In a gesture of equality, the theater paired my play with an autobiographical performance called *The Prostate Dialogues*, written by a very talented storyteller name John. I have to sit through my colleague's play to be a good theater person.

I slip into the second-floor balcony where I watch the same rude audience—those who remained—respond to my colleague's drama with deafening, frequent guffaws. I can see why too. John comes off as a lovable fellow simply telling the tale of how he found peace after his struggle. He is not the least bit freakish. He's not a broken little child.

After this second piece ends, amidst a roar of applause, I run back to the lobby. Aha, Kurt is waiting for me. I get that hug but his body feels stiff. Pulling away, he asks, "Do you have your things?"

I don't yet. I ramble about a bulky coat and a purse and some props and a bag of makeup. He tells me he's already packed up my video camera.

We're outside now and have hardly spoken. In the January chill, we scurry to our nest, thirty minutes by foot, our arms loaded with theater equipment. On 17th Street, we make a right. Restaurants line both sides of this wide road. Early in our dating history, Kurt and I sat by the window at the Turkish place trading secrets. More recently, we giggled over fat burgers and skinny fries at the newish wine bar a little up the road. I can't understand why he's not talking, but I can't take it anymore.

"Did you hate it?" I blurt out.

"Not hate . . ." His focus is on the pavement in front of him.

"I know. It was bad." In the silence that follows, I smell food from this block, all mixed up—Turkish fish, red meat, that herb they put in Pho that makes me ill. It's not the Pho, this time, that's making my stomach turn. "Was it that bad?" I ask.

"I can't believe you humiliated me," Kurt explodes into the air as if he's been holding this in for hours. I suppose he has.

"What?" I feel punched from behind.

He picks up his pace. "You publicly humiliated me." I watch the back of his leather jacket as he gets farther away from me.

"Would you slow down?" I shout.

"Sorry," he replies with a tight jaw, but he complies.

"*How* did I humiliate you?"

His eyes stay forward. "I asked you if I could read what you'd written, and you kept saying you would let me see it. But you didn't. People were laughing at me."

I stop dead. He does too. I'm trying to recollect what I wound up showing him—the first scene, for sure, and at least two others. We talked about the play though, a lot. But he's right. I never showed him the whole thing. I grab his arm. "They weren't laughing at you, Kurt. They were laughing at me. I'm the fuck-up."

"I can't believe I trusted you," he says, charging beyond me again. Then he elaborates, with a cracked voice. It's the same sentiment over and over: betrayal, boundaries, and no privacy. "How can I ever trust you?" he says right outside our apartment.

All this effort to be unbroken and, look at me, I just broke the foundation of my marriage.

Tips for *Your* Pleasure Plan

Something to Try:

Challenge your shame for a day. Choose something specific you're ashamed of with regard to your erotic self. It could be connected to your body, your sexual history, or something else. Behave for a day as if you're not ashamed. Whom will you talk to? Where will you go? What will you do? Think of your whole day as a mini-experiment.

Journal Prompts:

1. Most of us could use self-forgiveness for something we're holding against ourselves. What do you need to forgive yourself for?

   _____

   _____

   _____

2. How would others benefit if you forgave yourself?

   _____

   _____

   _____

3. How would your life be different if you forgave yourself?

   _____

   _____

   _____

11

The Hospital

Right after the play, my pelvic pain spreads so that it's no longer confined to coitus. It becomes a 24/7 ache that's migrated from the genitals, north, settling right around my rib cage. Once upon a time—upon meeting a blond date in a French restaurant—this area of the body whispered to me, *I like him.* Now I can't decipher what my torso is communicating.

I do not tell Kurt about my distress. Too much weight has fallen upon his shoulders in the last five weeks—since our fight walking home from the theater. First, he retreated to an emotional cave featuring electronic devices and excess beer. He claimed it was the only way to process what I'd done. Then his best friend Scott went into hospice, only months after his initial cancer diagnosis. Finally, ten days ago, Kurt's father passed away. My loving father-in-law was ninety-six years old, with a history of recent strokes, so his death was not unexpected. Still, my husband is devastated. We just got back from the funeral in Indiana.

Now, Kurt is sighing a lot with eyes vacant or full of water. Most nights he turns his back to me as soon as we get under the covers as if my touch is a megaton mass overloading his fragility. Often, when

I wake up to pee, I discover him in the living room, staring into the harsh, dim light of his cell phone, or he's sobbing. How can I burden this man with my stomachache?

I mean, is it even physical? I too am mourning the death of my father-in-law. When I married Kurt, miraculously, I had a dad again—a healthy one. Al was an upright, laughing soul who once gave me a turquoise ring belonging to his recently departed wife, Kurt's mom. Losing him hollowed me out as if the grim reaper spared my life but scooped out my viscera with his scythe. It's the same doubled-over weakness I felt when my own parents died. My gut is surely in loss mode, but it's compounding an underlying brokenness: what never got resolved through *The* (now-defunct) *Pleasure Plan*. Whatever the source, I'm determined to spare Kurt my irksome complications.

Yet, after a week of torment—eventually conquering a huge swath of me, from bra line to crotch—I'm forced to confess what's going on.

"Your alarm," Kurt croaks that Wednesday morning as we both cringe from the buzzer's volume.

"I know," I reply. But shutting it off would mean rolling over, which might aggravate the burning. In the last few days, the emptiness in my stomach has been permeated with fire.

"Are you sick?" my husband asks from his half of the bed. He scoots in closer. Sometimes I call him The Radiator because of the heat his skin emits, especially under our duvet. I usually love it, as a person who's frequently cold, but now it makes me feel feverish.

"Yeah," I reply, running my tongue around my mouth where it detects a vague but vile taste. "I think I have a stomach thing."

"Yeesh."

"Yeesh."

Kurt gets out of bed and I watch him. His arms reach to the ceiling.

A knee bends, then the other. He told me a few days ago he'd try battling his sadness by waking up with more deliberate energy. And my husband always does what he says. If I ask him to pick up extra-soft toilet paper on sale, a light bulb for the fridge, and a bagel with tomato slices, he'll return with all three, plus yummy chocolate for me. In contrast, I'll forget the bulb and the bagel. Exercises complete, Kurt is next to me again, hot hand on my forehead. "You think it's a bug?" he guesses. If I say yes, he'll run to CVS for Imodium, whatever I need.

But I don't think *bug* is exactly right.

I can't rule it out, though. I've been too busy—no, scared—to acknowledge *what's actually taking place in my body*. I inhale deeply as my heart flaps its wings like a hummingbird. I tentatively press my lower abdomen, noticing the right side is excruciatingly tender. The sensation is familiar, though. Blessedly. It feels like ovulation. Severe ovulation. Wasn't Tamar talking recently about periods? Hers have become heavy and painful due to over-forty hormone flux. *My hormones must be in flux*, I think as I start doing math. The last time I got my period was two weeks ago. Before that, a month before. I'm still regular. Still, I'm forty-eight and a half. Isn't menopause around the corner? Maybe it's already here. "It's *not* a bug. You know what this is? It's menopause," I tell my husband.

Then I tell everyone!

While getting my teeth cleaned later that morning, after having the hygienist adjust the chair three times because the angle is bothering my middle, I confide in this oral-health maven, who already expressed compassion with her gentle scaling, that my difficulty is related to "the saga of menopause." She gives me a knowing wink.

In the afternoon, I inform six adult students who signed up for my storytelling workshop that I may not be my best because of "annoying estrogen depletion." They chuckle. Kurt didn't when I used the same phrase on him an hour prior. While he was driving me here, I asked him to pull over so I could vomit in the street.

After the class, I repeat my malaise to Scott's mother. We have come to our friend's charming DC apartment—Kurt, me, and Scott's parents—to empty it, now that he's gone into hospice. *He is never coming back.* I sit on the hardwood floor, propped against a couch that will be donated. Scared of passing out, I stay put. The whole time, I'm afraid Scott's Midwestern matriarch will think I'm lazy for not lifting boxes or carrying furniture into the basement. After all, *she's* doing these things, even though she's in her eighties and losing her son to cancer, even though she's a cancer survivor herself. "I'm having menopause issues," I reveal as a way to bond with her, crone to crone. "Oh Boy!" she says with a sympathetic roll of her eyes.

Ultimately, I tell myself that vanishing menses—and related, weird ovulation—are the source of my trouble. *Ovulation only lasts a day,* I chant to myself at home as I make up the couch so I don't disrupt Kurt's sleep.

As soon as I slip under the covers, I enter hell. Purpose-driven devils are poking me from the inside with searing spears. I try to sleep by putting on a nightgown and taking it off, by slipping into socks and removing them. Remarkably, I nod off.

At three in the morning, my eyelids pop open. My body is blanched in lucid terror—*something is terribly wrong.* Still, I wait. Why should worn-out Kurt forgo slumber? Perhaps I'm still hoping my affliction will resolve on its own so I won't have to face misguided, malevolent doctors. It doesn't resolve, of course. As soon as I hear Kurt's alarm go off, at 6 AM, I burst into the bedroom to say what I've been rehearsing for hours, "I need to go to the emergency room."

Kurt springs into action with twelve arms. My husband, who has been mad and distant and grieving for weeks, boils water for tea, helps me put on clothes, and pulls the car around.

Since we arrive at the ER around seven, and only a handful of people are seated, I'm thinking a diagnosis will be quick. But hours course by with many tests yet only speculation—ectopic pregnancy, appendicitis, or bowel obstruction. It's like a mini-version of my project. I'm seeing doctor after doctor, and they can't figure out what's wrong with me. Until Dr. Lee arrives.

At 3 PM, eight hours after I entered this hospital, Dr. Lee, a Chinese-American surgeon with a long, regal neck and short, clean nails, comes to my stretcher in the hall. She smells like expensive soap, not just the hand sanitizer everyone uses around here. Taking my hand, gazing deeply into my eyes, she discloses that my appendix ruptured two days before. At the point of bursting, I should have been screaming in agony, according to this physician.

"You must have a really high tolerance for pain," she remarks with a little laugh meant to put me at ease. It doesn't. Because I waited so long to seek medical help, a local infection has spread to my upper and lower intestines. She begins drawing me a picture on the back of a prescription pad. If I hadn't delayed, explains the kind-eyed surgeon, she'd have performed a routine appendectomy. Now she can't operate. All she can do is give me antibiotics to, hopefully, stop the infection from taking over my body. Otherwise, she'll need to start cutting out organs.

Immediately I go numb as if "cutting out organs" is an angry boy who pushed me into a pool of freezing water. Coming up for air, an image flashes across my inner eyes. It's startling in its un-sexiness. "Could I end up with a colostomy bag?" I ask.

"Yes, but that's not our worry right now," says the woman who has put down the drawing so she can pick up my cold hand again. I don't want her to ever let go. "What we need to watch out for is sepsis," she explains. "Do you know what sepsis is?"

I nod. I've seen it on the TV news, some special report. It's an out-of-control bacterial disaster that often leads to death. From the bottom of me, a stick of dynamite explodes debris that's been blocking clear thinking for a solid week, maybe forever. "I could die?" I ask.

"Yes," she answers. "But let's not go there."

Where else is there to go?

The next thing I know, they are wheeling my gurney through halls and elevators so they can admit me, indefinitely. *How could I do this to myself? How could I be so stupid?* They deliver me to a room, hooking me up with my new lover, a morphine pump. My eyes go wet with gratitude. I can't believe the throbbing has stopped. But my comprehension will not be subdued. I won't let it. I have to figure out how to save my life.

For the next twenty-four hours, except for trips to the bathroom, I'm immobile. Even shallow breathing hurts. This gives me time to reflect. What about the months I just spent studying the art of healing? After gynecology, and vaginal weights, and hypnosis, and tantra, and EMDR, and EFT, and trauma therapy, and more, have I uncovered anything useful? Any recovery knowledge I might apply to this predicament?

Perhaps I don't need my own wisdom because Dr. Lee has a strategy for getting me out of here—her own Plan. It involves this IV pole I'm now married to. One mainline is for high-gear antibiotics. Another is for fluids. A third is my inaccessible opiate paramour (I have to press a button to get more, but only after I'm in awful distress). Repairing me is also the starchy blue gown with snaps in the back for easy prodding; a mechanical bed with white flat sheets that don't stay flat; and a nubby blanket so thin it seems disposable. There's the stench of disinfectant and relentless beeps. My insurance pays for everything—a situation not to be taken for granted in this country—so these *accoutrements* must be the best offered. They are what will mend me.

No, that's wrong. Only my own red blood cells can perform that task, by conquering their white cousins. *How can I get them to do their job?* For those first twenty-four hours, my brain buzzes around the universe, despite my immobility, searching for an answer. Meanwhile, flesh-eating bacteria have their way with me. At the end of that full day, I'm convinced I do not have the wherewithal to heal. These secrets are utterly beyond me.

Then they wheel in Jennifer.

Jennifer reminds me of a young woman I knew in college that we all described as *a waif*. She described herself that way too. My new roommate is similar in her aloof gaze; small bones; and straight, fine brown hair. She now occupies the bed next to mine, closest to our bathroom and window. At first, when I try to chat with her, Jennifer provides single-word answers. She also complains to the nurse that I make too much noise when I use the bathroom. But a day into our living arrangement, she shares with me that she's a thirty-two-year-old proofreader with her own mysterious pelvic pain. In fact, this is her third hospitalization for the same ailment because, so far, none have been able to cure her.

Relief might be more complicated than she recognizes.

That night, while eavesdropping on a call between her and another, whom I speculate is the handsome young man with dreadlocks who came to see her that afternoon, I find out Jennifer was molested as a child. Tearfully, she says into the receiver, "Something happened to me when I was a kid.... My parents don't even know." Overhearing her situation is like looking into a fun house mirror, but which of us is distorted? Naturally, I think it's her.

For three days, swarms of attending physicians, residents, interns, and medical students (this is a teaching hospital) descend upon my roommate. The species are differentiated: gynecology, gastroenterology, psychiatry, social work, hepatology, and urology. At every encounter, a doctor asks Jennifer to rate her pain on a scale of one to ten. She always declares "nine." The minute they leave, she grabs her cell phone to complain about what just occurred. Then she picks up the landline and orders a tuna sandwich with chips and a diet coke. She does this while twirling her hair or the constantly tangled phone cord.

Untangling *her* becomes my obsession.

She is a tight ball of complications but I recognize some yarn: a heart with holes eaten out of it, parents consumed with illness or home renovations, the shock of selfish cocks. But what if this collection of scars is wrapped around a transformative, hard gem? A philosopher's stone. In alchemy, a philosopher's stone is a magical object or substance that can turn ordinary metal to gold. Or in this case, sickness to health. If I can discover her alchemizing force, mine might be nearby—in my adjacent bed. Then I'd know how to fix my infection and other brokenness.

Every day, Kurt comes before and after work, bringing me gifts like kombucha, a stuffed tiger, or a squishy elephant to help me maintain arm strength. That night I ask him to bring me *The Pleasure Plan* journal. I begin jotting down Jennifer's interactions. Snippets are audible, even when they close the curtain to examine her. I note what her docs suspect, telephone play-by-plays, and lots of tuna.

Meanwhile, my white blood cell count stays dangerously high, and my own medical team has no solutions other than to wait and see if I can conquer these bacteria. When they ask me to estimate my level of pain, I never go above a five—despite being splayed out like a blaze victim because even blinking hurts. This is *with* morphine.

On my fourth day tied to tubes, my pen witnesses a notable change in my roommate. She is giving a person on the other end of the phone an ultimatum. It's probably the boy with dreadlocks. "If you don't want to be my friend, then don't," she seethes in a half-whisper. "I didn't tell you to come here, you know. And if you're not going to believe me, then don't come here, okay? Because I'm not crazy." Then she is shrieking, "I'm not crazy. I'm not crazy!"

If I weren't a puffy zombie I would jump up and hug her. Of course, she's not crazy. She's just stuck, like all of us who've been harmed by pigs and happenstance. We are trapped, replicating horror in perpetuity. It's wired in. As far back as I can remember, I've known about this permanence. I think of my mom and her neurological rainstorms.

Every time a downpour came through, my mother would take my brother and me into the shadowy living room of our old house, where lightning and thunder turned the sky violent. We'd take Mom's lead, pushing palms against our ears so we wouldn't hear the threat.

"It's not bombs," my mother would say, "it sounds like bombs, but it's not bombs." Though just a kid, it was obvious to me she was trying to get out of a maze. The first time I chanted yoga mantras, the sound made me think of the low-pitched, hypnotizing drone in my mother's voice as she repeated over and over, "It's not bombs, but it sounds like bombs." She wanted her brain to retain a fact her body could not—that she *wasn't* being attacked. I grew up believing a body under siege could never believe in a new, safe reality.

But deep in my ventricles, I carve out hope for Jennifer because I want to create hope for myself. As I fall asleep that night, a prayer nestles in my chest until it delivers me to a Caribbean beach and the warm sea. I'm swimming with my mother and also Jennifer, but then they're gone. It's just me diving under with legs kicking vigorously. In real life, I've never been a good swimmer. Here, my muscles have the grace and force I experience on the stage. My thighs push against the resistance of the current. There's no narrative to this part of the nightscape, only travel through an undersea world that's sun-soaked green, perfectly clear, and pleasing.

I'm still primarily in my dream as I open my eyes with a grin. Surrounding me is the same wet warmth of the ocean. Slowly, I grasp why—my hospital gown . . . the sheets . . . the blanket . . . are soiled. There is a foul odor. I continue to soil the bed. I have lost control of my bowels.

Yelling for help is mandatory, yet humiliation closes my windpipe. I don't know how to have this kind of need. My face is tomato red, sweating: *I must not go above five in my pain. I must not go above five.* I don't say it to myself. I don't have to. It's so ingrained.

No, Jennifer is not the distorted human. I am. I'm the one lying in her own shit.

In lieu of assistance, I swing my legs over the bed and stand up. I need to protect the floor, so I strip my bed and stuff it—sheets and blanket—between my legs. Thusly encumbered, I unplug the IV pole and find a clean robe, some underwear. I shuffle with this bundle to the bathroom, quietly, so as not to wake Jennifer. After showering and putting on clean garb, I somehow find fresh linens I put on the mattress, defecating the whole time.

Then I get back into bed.

Realizing I'm in the same predicament, I start sobbing, sound-lessly. But just as the first wave subsides, I discover my philosopher's stone. It drops down from the sky. Or falls out of my very active ass. It's true I need healing, of ravenous bacteria and terror tucked into the folds of my labia. But underlying everything that's wrong with me is the exact same brokenness. To fix myself—to escape my own maze—I don't need healing at all. What I need is a *nine* on my pain scale.

I cry out, "Nurse! Nurse!! I NEED A DIAPER."

What I need is power.

Tips for *Your* Pleasure Plan

Something to Try:

While at work or doing something busy, set an alarm for twenty-five minutes. When the alarm goes off, ask yourself what your body needs right then. Spend five minutes giving your body what it asks for. Repeat this cycle throughout the day.

FYI: This is an adaptation of the Pomodoro Technique developed by Francesco Cirillo (see the Appendix for details).

Journal Prompts:

1. Are you able to hear your body talking to you about your needs? Do you know when you're hungry? Thirsty? Tired? Experiencing a full belly? Have an urge to use the bathroom?

   _____

   _____

   _____

2. If you're not able to hear your body talking to you regarding one or more areas, how can you fine-tune this "hearing"?

   _____

   _____

   _____

3. If you're able to hear your body, how do you respond? With dismissal? Attentiveness? Frustration? Compassion?

   _____

   _____

   _____

Part 3
Advanced Studies in Pleasure

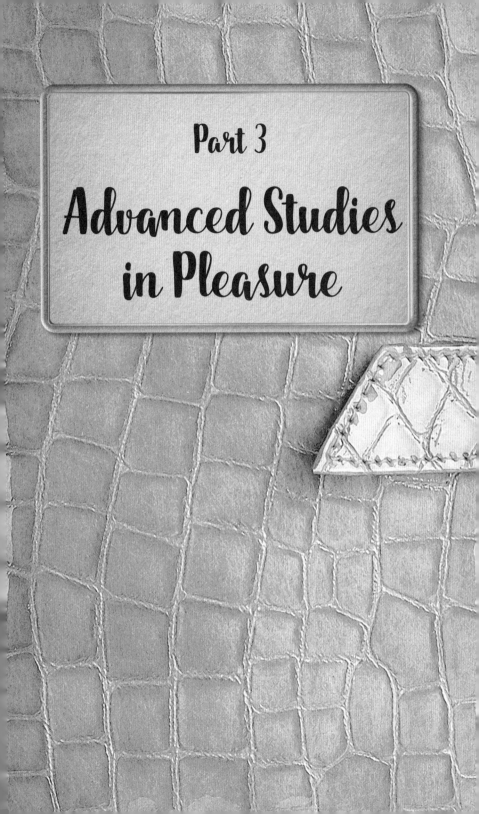

12

Recovery

Look Ma, no colostomy bag!

Even so, much has transpired in the last six months. First, my immune system crushed the infection. It took a week of hospitalization, but I got to keep my organs (fist pump). There *was* aftermath, though. Hot throbbing viscera required eight weeks to chill. Only then was I cleared for appendectomy. The operation was successful, but I needed more months to allay disturbed tissue again. During this long restorative time, I was not to engage in intercourse—special orders from Dr. Lee. It made sense: Where would Kurt's tumescence fit amidst my own swollen organs?

I was glad to have this dedicated half-year for mending. It felt like respect. Kurt was respecting my convalescence, and I was respecting the power commitment I'd made in the hospital—to voice my corporeal needs. I'm listening to my body now, hearing her response.

But now the six months are up.

I'm cleared to merge sheath and sword, to reexplore the betterment of bonking. Here's the thing though: I'm really digging celibacy. Having Kurt want nothing more from my evenings than shared viewing of Jeopardy is fab. Feet on my husband's lap, I reach forward to tickle his arm. He purrs like a handsome, tamed Tabby. Later, there might be a bit of oral:

"Can you hand me a fork near the stove?"

"Oh, I'll give you a fork, all right."

"I know you will!"

After the couples retreat, we ramped up this repartee so we'd be "making love" all the time, which we are.

Except we're not.

As much as I enjoy flirting, I'm also an untrampled forest hiding out in my own woods. It's peaceful but dark. Darkness born of skepticism. I don't know what is possible for me anymore. I wait for Kurt to suggest a "rendezvous," pulling me out into the sun. Weirdly, he doesn't. In fact, rather than extend suggestive jokes, pushing for concrete where's and when's, my spouse starts sleeping on the couch. He says it's because of insomnia.

Lonely in our double bed, I'm convinced we're replicating my parents' marriage—and I'm responsible. As far back as my memory goes, Mom and Dad slept in separate rooms. My mother said it was because my dad snored. But I suspected it was because of his neurological disease. She was no longer attracted to him. Or maybe it was another situation. Mom's first husband, Max, had been "a sex maniac." She only mentioned him once, when I was in my twenties, but she told me everything. He wanted intercourse several times a day. They were only married a few months when she left him. "I couldn't take it," she relayed to me with face contorted and hands on her hair. "Feh," she said, mock spitting but really meaning it. After she divorced him, Max stalked my mother in the New York City subway. She'd be traveling to work, at the bottom of the stairs, about to go through the turnstile, when she'd see him lurking in a shadowy patch between the token booth and wall. She pretended not to notice as she rushed through the pokey metal bars. She knew she wasn't safe.

I do not want my mother's relationship with Max, or my dad. After two weeks of marriage-room divide, I give Kurt a palm of Melatonin. "Schmookie, come to bed," I beg. "You need a full night's rest." He takes the pills but says, "I can't sleep there!"

That weekend I find out why. That weekend, while my honey and I stroll through an apple orchard on a sweatery fall day, he says, "I think it's depression." Kids with faces as red as the fruit in their hands, dash around us. Kurt continues, "Everything is ... flat." Then he ticks off contributing factors: Scott's decline, his father's death, work-related issues, the stress of my illness. The humiliation of my theater endeavor.

My heart shatters from being on this list. Spiderweb cracks spread throughout my chest. Some fractures are comprised of guilt, but others are pure panic. Depression was the name eventually given to my father's isolation and pessimism. After Dad's passing, I asked a social worker at the nursing home where he ended up to diagnose him, posthumously. I never had language for his strange behavior. *What was wrong with him?*

"If I had to guess," offered this hazel-eyed professional, whose name was also Laura, "I'd say he had an anxiety-based depression, probably his whole life."

I'm not worried about Kurt having this same diagnosis; as I write this, 80 percent of my friends are currently popping a Prozac, a Xanax, or both. I'm scared of the psychological stench in my home that emanated from my father's sickness. Every time Dad yelled at the television from his room, or mumbled to himself, or drank out of the milk container, my mother would twirl a finger next to her temple, making a *loco* circle—all behind his back. "See? He's mentally ill," she'd say to my brother and me. After immense suffering, she was stuck with a husband who couldn't take care of her. She'd gotten a bum rap.

A lemon.

Her bitterness is what terrifies me.

But in the orchard, watching parents control their children, who are frenzied with apple abundance, I'm inspired to control *myself*—the way I handle my spouse's condition. Also, Kurt is nothing like my dad, who wouldn't see a doctor for his ailments (his doc-phobia might have been worse than my mom's). In contrast, my husband is already inching ahead. By the time we leave the grove, Kurt has googled and found a psychiatrist he'd like to see—a well-regarded friend of a friend.

Before he can get his appointment, though, Kurt slips deeper into blackness. This time, he doesn't sleep for five nights in a row. On the sixth day he skips work, spending hours on the floor, mostly hugging his knees. When he tries expressing his feelings, he beats himself with his hands. "I hate my life," he sobs. "I hate myself. I hate my life."

I sit on the rug with him, stroking his hair. Diana's words at the couples retreat float into my thoughts—"Don't wait until your beloved is dying to give him your loving attention." I ponder: *How much of partnership is not only gifting focus to our partner before he dies but helping this person stay alive?* Fundamentally, isn't this what marriage is? Foundationally, isn't this love?

I think of Mom and her friend Rivka. In the last days of the war, the two of them were infected with typhus in a fetid concentration camp on the Baltic Sea. The Nazis were losing their territory in Poland so they decided to "liquidate" this camp, marching thousands of half-dead prisoners to Germany, which was hundreds of miles away. The journey launched in the forest, where Rivka stumbled immediately.

A German shepherd savagely bit her leg. My mother pulled her friend up. "You have to keep walking," she pleaded with Rivka. "If you fall again, they'll shoot you. Just lean here," she said, supporting Rivka's weight against a hip that had no flesh on it. "See? ... Keep walking. I love you. I love you."

"I love you," I say to Kurt, massaging lavender oil into his temples. "I love you."

I want to think this helps. Either way, slowly but steadily, my husband climbs out of his steep well of sadness. Once he finds ground, he dedicates himself to dopamine, the neurotransmitter producing light in the eyes and lightness in the soul. He dedicates himself to curing what underlies his woes too—mostly, a general sense of powerlessness and constant self-incrimination. He is the one on a healing odyssey now. And it's impressive: weekly shrink appointments, an online happiness course, meditation, Prozac, Wellbutrin, mindfulness, Buddhism, coffee with friends, journaling in the morning, and tons of veggies.

Watching his determined march toward joy, I reflect upon the inertia of my own recovery. What's at the heart of it? Definitely cynicism—but perhaps it's also dopamine (or the lack thereof). When I ended my repair adventure, my boudoir experience was less than jaunty. In other words, I wasn't loving lovemaking enough to long for it, or even repair it. And now that Kurt is getting better, we've started screwing again—yup, status quo. So why not discover a way to enjoy it more?

The science is clear on this. Kurt's happiness course has taught *me* so much as well. Dopamine is most elevated in anticipation of pleasure, more than during the act itself—as long as the last experience was awesome. Dopamine is our natural motivator.

Making sex great is what will inspire me to want sex. In other words, I'm right back where I started—not knowing how to improve my sensual experience. How do I change my circumstance, once and for all?

One afternoon, around this time, as my honey sits in our living room watching joy videos on his laptop, I open my matching computer, turning to my play, *Married Sex*. Where did this material end up? Did I uncover anything I might apply as propulsion? I did! It's not in the play though; it's in a Panera. That's where I originally spoke to that sex therapist. Her recommendation is the one loose end I never tied up through my theater project. I was too freaked out by the call and didn't have time to un-freak out. But now I do.

Written down in *The Pleasure Plan* journal, which I fetch, is what the sex therapist said. Minutes later, I arrive at this passage: "I send all my pelvic-pain patients to physical therapy." She gave me the names of three specialists, which I'm staring at right now. Obviously, it's time to resurrect my quest. *The Pleasure Plan 2.0*. The thought makes the floorboards quake, or that's my thighs, because I no longer have a deadline, or Shirley, or Ari—so no accountability. Can I just proceed? Can I trust myself to march forward?

Of the three physical therapists, I choose Stephanie. She practices at a facility that is close to my house. On the way over, passing calla lilies that have spring-like blooms in September, my eyes mist because, although I've been trying varied betterment techniques, I've yet to have someone directly treat the body part actually abused. In a vague way, that's what I had wanted from the Tantrika. I think of ancient days. When a young girl was violated, did the midwives come 'round? Did they place hands on this child's tiny mound, to bring healing. Maybe they applied poultices of chamomile, myrrh, and sage.

When I get to the doctor's office, I discover it's more beige than sage. Corporate bland permeates carpet, wallpaper, counter, and vinyl chairs I do not sit in. Instead, I stand agape at what is in front of me—a glass partition. On the other side, an elderly guy in baggy gym trunks and sports shirt is on the matted floor, rolling his torso over a foam roller. Massage tables are in open view. A teenage boy is having his knee manipulated by a dude who resembles Tony Robbins.

Is this where Stephanie will be tutoring my vagina? I'm about to find out. A woman is approaching me, arms swinging. "Laura?"

"Hi."

Her jeans, gray-streaked-brown hair, and John Lennon glasses remind me of cool moms I knew in the seventies. I adored hugging those women, who sometimes gave me cookies. Stephanie takes me through a hallway running along the glass divider. On the left side of this corridor are private rooms, I discover. Our room has baby-blue walls and two framed posters of abstract artwork, mostly colorful swirls.

Things happen quickly after I put my bag down. We chat a while; I undress from the waist down; Stephanie gives me a white hand towel to cover my pudendum. As I lie back with my legs in a butterfly pose like during the yoni massage, cold air blows from a vent but I'm not chilly. Proud heat is rising from my body. *I'm getting treated for vaginismus.* I don't know why it's taken me this long, but I'm here now—with agency.

That doesn't mean this feels good. Butt cheeks lift off the table, legs twist, breath pushes through gritted teeth while I try to stay still. "Is it bad?" I ask the vagina whisperer.

"Not the worst I've seen, but yeah. It's bad."

But she's getting to the bottom of things. I learn a ton. Vaginismus is extreme tightness of the muscles controlling the pelvic floor. Simultaneously, incongruously, it's also extreme weakness of these same muscles, and spasm is common. Also, this set of muscles can be implicated in a variety of disorders, like incontinence and weakness after pregnancy. When I tell Stephanie about the little weights Dr. Graham, the gynecologist, prescribed, the PT shakes her John Lennon glasses from side to side, "No! No! No!" she says. "Your muscles don't know how to relax! We can't start building strength until we teach them to let go."

Her passion for my process brings contraction to another part of me. In the back of my throat, a little dam is holding back thirty years of tears. "Thank you for finally clearing this up," I tell her.

"You're welcome," she responds. But then she bites her lip. "You have something besides vaginismus, though. Did anybody ever tell you?"

"*Another* vagina thing?"

"No, this is outside the vagina. It's called vestibulitis."

I'm utterly perplexed. But she uncovers a burning mystery. Vestibulitis is causing these sensations. It's overactive nerves in the vestibule, which is the area inside the inner lips, but *outside* the vagina. Luckily, she thinks the kind of vestibulitis I have can be remedied the same way as vaginismus—with weekly PT and daily Kegels, which I'll be able to commence once the tightness dissipates a little. Stephanie also wants me to use the dilators three times a week. These are the "sex toys" I thought I'd be using when I first found out about vaginismus.

In fact, I had bought these rocket-shaped insertion tools once I started *The Pleasure Plan*. I just never used them after my awful experience with the vaginal weights. I stuffed the dilators in the same drawer as the little tortures.

But when I get home from my appointment with Stephanie that

day, I fish them out. The kit has five phallic-shaped cylinders. The largest of these hollow faux fornicators is the width and height of an average man's member—apparently 6 inches long and 1.5 inches in diameter, according to the tape measure I use on this thing. The other four dildos decrease in height and girth until we reach the smallest, the size of an average index finger—3 inches long and 0.5 inches in diameter. Also included in the kit is a single Q-tip, hygienically wrapped in plastic. This is in case the first trainer is still uncomfortable. After trial and error, I choose one of the middle sizes. I'm to push this plastic in and out of me for fifteen minutes. My toes curl in dread. *Who is designing these un-lusty tools?*

Kurt is in the next room retraining his brain for happiness, so I retrain too.

Not just that day, but going forward.

After three weeks of in-office massage and at-home dilator action, after an intercourse pause to make sure my inner muscles don't revert to old patterns, I start improving. That's what Stephanie thinks.

At a session around this time, she pats my instep, which is near the hooha opening she's just entered. "You're doing great," she says with a smile, revealing dimples. I hadn't noticed the dimples. After maneuvers, as she's washing her hands, I work up the courage to ask this: "So what *should* sex feel like?"

Stephanie closes the tap and tilts her salt-and-pepper hair. She's glancing into the distance, toward one of the posters on the wall, an abstract print with coils of red and black. After another moment, she replies, "Actually... it's kind of boring."

I laugh, but it's more like a burp of surprise. Surely she's joking, but I don't think she is. Standing closer to my table now with her chin tucked in, she peers at me, mascara to mascara. These are the serious secrets of women. My heart sinks, almost to the area she was just releasing. *Is this what's on the other side of my randy rainbow?*

But then I mentally scan the stack of shagging books on my bedside table. Many quote the same statistic: only 30 percent of females have orgasms through penetration alone; another 30 percent need simultaneous clitoral stimulation; and the last third do not climax through penetration at all. As my physical therapist tidies up, I surmise she must be a person whose boat is not rocked by cock, or other kinds of insertion. If I can get my vaginismus solved, I'm curious what group *I'll* belong to.

I'm closing in on this reveal. Allowed to have coitus again, I find it uncomfortable but not nearly as much, especially with techniques Stephanie passed on. Upon entry, I "pump" my Kegel apparatus to find neutral, that is, a state of non-spasm I can control. Then the fun begins. Madame releases as Monsieur enters; and she holds him tight as he exits. In essence, Stephanie taught me the "Intro to Fucking for Physicians" course I was hoping my gynecologist would have passed on to me. It's not my gyno's fault she lacked this education. I've recently discovered most doctors—including gynecologists and urologists—only receive *one day* of human sexuality curricula during their years of medical school and residency.

Regardless, my squeezebox is getting less squeezed. Remarkably. But for how long?

Despite tangible improvement between the sheets, I'm having trouble believing in a lasting cure. I call Wendy, who began dilator use around the same time for her own vaginismus, discovered through my project. She's fine now. I scrutinize Kurt, who is, undeniably, better. I even begin physical therapy on another body part, my weak left shoulder. Same facility; different therapist. I'm trying to trust this process—rewiring through repetition. The zeitgeist is buzzing with examples of this, of *neuroplasticity*. It's physical therapy and Cognitive Behavioral Therapy. It's affirmations and Prolonged Exposure.

And yet, when it comes to my own renewal, I can't obliterate those damn bombs in my mother's living room. The explosions she swore by, even though it was just rainstorms. Her nervous system drew a line between boom and bomb. Full stop. That's how trauma works! Or so I always thought. I've been so convinced that it's permanent. The data backs me up, though. At the military trauma conference I attended, I became aware that some studies show two-thirds of PTSD patients are incurable, despite all the fab methods touted at the conference.

There's another wrench thrown into my box as well. It concerns the reason my mother was exposed to bombs in the first place. After holding Rivka up on that death march, my mother and other prisoners were loaded onto a barge taken out to the Baltic Sea. It was immediately shelled by the English. At first, Mom went below-deck, but a lascivious man was leering and he might have touched her. This was another prisoner, tortured and starved for years, barely alive, but his dick was apparently working. My mother told me she was scared of being raped. So she went to the upper deck—where there was a greater risk of dying.

These threats, I believe, were linked for Mom. Merged together, they connect the two of us—her fear of rape on one end, and my experience of being raped during sex on the other. A single circuit uniting us.

But then, on a miraculous evening, this line is severed.

For the first time in my life, I do not feel assaulted as I make love. It's Wednesday, at seven in the evening. An ordinary night with two candles lit and French music playing on Pandora, yet what ensues is absolutely wacko. I mean, *is this my genitalia?* To be honest, some mini-demons do make an appearance between my thighs, a twinge or two, but I scare them off with my new yoni power. Consequently, I am able to lose myself, modestly. Then it's over.

After hugging my guy, I bounce my bottom on the bed like it's a trampoline, to celebrate. We pour glasses of wine and sip it with our pinkies out. Yet privately, I cogitate on what was missing. What about undulations and juicy transcendence? How about moaning on the mountaintop? Because mostly what I experienced was...pressure.

In other words, Stephanie was right. Sex *is* kind of boring.

But I think I know why.

I write it out in my Pleasure journal the next morning. Here's the thing: I've been so focused on vag function, I haven't yet cultivated the erotic universe *inside me.* I've breathed in its external fragrance, but have no idea what entices my heart and groin to engage in physical love, or what might provide ecstasy. However, if I got this far, then maybe I *do* believe in new circuitry—even for survivors like myself. At least, this is what I want to hope. But where to start? My pleasure wiring is either nonexistent or terribly installed.

There's a simple remedy, though, that's not simple in the least.

If I crave ecstasy, I need to go through every single sex wire in my nervous system and replace it. Stephanie cannot do this for me. Nor can a hypnotist, or a trauma therapist, or anyone that's not me.

How will I know how to locate each synapsis to correct it?

I don't know!

But I have to find out.

Tips for *Your* Pleasure Plan

Something to Try:

To rewire your brain, recognize a pattern in your life. Then do something different! Choose another place to eat lunch, a new street for getting to work, a different pen to write with. Continue with this new pattern, noticing how long it takes for it to become rote. Keep this updated pattern or start a new one.

And, on a related topic, if dilators are part of your sexual healing see the Recommended Resources section in the Appendix for information about these.

Journal Prompts:

1. Who inspires you to move forward when you get stuck?

   _____

   _____

   _____

2. How does this person keep faith or recover from failure?

   _____

   _____

   _____

3. What can you learn from this person about power and/or resilience?

   _____

   _____

   _____

13

Ah, Look at All the Shiny Women

I start with feathers—blazing pink ones, peacock size. They're all over the lobby of this theater, resting on registration tables, tucked into waistbands, and palmed by va-va-voom volunteers, who wear black tees. The pink lettering on these shirts says, "8000 Nerve Endings." I think this refers to the clitoris. The seminar I'm attending this weekend, led by a famous woman named Mama Gena, focuses on female rapture. If I want new circuitry, comprehensively, why not connect it to pleasure? Pleasure as a generator or power station—or its own electromagnetic system. You know how some techies make sure everything in their homes—from lamps to alarms to toilets—connects to Wi-Fi? Pink nerve endings could be my Wi-Fi. As I make my way from the lobby to the theater itself, two feather-bearing femmes frame me in the doorway, running their sensual plumes down my body.

My updated life is anointed.

Claiming a chair in this hall is not easy. Though there are many rows of velvet, rose-colored seats, similar to an old movie theater, most are taken. The place is packed with hundreds of chatting, dancing, whispering, and mirth-making women. By appearances, some have a Harley waiting for them outside. Others have a chauffeur; a magical tree; a boyfriend on a leash; or no one because her companion is right here, a book in her oversized bag. Perhaps, I'm being typecast as well in my navy knit dress, black cardigan, black scarf, and snow-stained wedge boots. My category might be called Wears-Too-Many-Layers. By the time I find a place near the back wall, I have forgotten the factions. We are a united mass of joie-seekers. We're even beginning to look the same. Every chair dons a gratis bubble-gum hued boa. I put mine on without hesitation, and feel like weeping—in relief and embarrassment, in camaraderie—because every woman in this room wants to be desirous.

I first heard of Mama Gena, and her School of Womanly Arts, from my friend Claire, who took several of this teacher's "expensive-but-incredible programs." Claire told me this guru, whose real name is Regena Thomashauer, is masterful at awakening the sexual energy of her participants. My buddy also mentioned that Mama Gena holds a free event in New York every year. To that, I said, *Hell Yes*, and now I'm about to meet the star.

Just then, a Goth-chic organizer jumps on the stage. "Are you ready to turn on?" she yells in her short, black dress and tall heels. She's making circles in front of her crotch. "Are you ready to turn on you-know-what?"

"Turn on the pussy," enthuses a muscle mama in a tutu to my right. She must be around eighty. "Turn on the pussy," she shouts again.

"Yes!!!" scream dedicated fans. It feels like most of the room has been here before.

"Ladies," bellows the announcer, "I bring you Mama Genaaaaaah." Music pounds, African drums, and here she comes. Well, only her feet. She's up in the air, horizontal, being carried by an all-male crew, who might have been recruited from a PTA gathering, a chorus casting call, and a plumber's union Meetup. As she floats down the aisle, above our crowns, I see pointy, patent-leather pumps... then long, tan legs... a torso snug in a wrap dress... and finally, a blond head of blown-out hair. I clap and boogie in my chair along with the throng because it's fun to be a groupie, even though I know so little about this woman.

I'm about to discover more.

Once Mama Gena is vertical, and the carriers have left—no boys allowed!—I am taken by Thomashauer's charged presence, lovely face, and her moxie. She strikes me as the kind of friend who would listen with nods as you complained about a salesperson at Macy's that wouldn't let you return a blouse. Then, she'd march to the store with you, arm-in-arm, getting those coins returned. I get this impression from how she refers to us. Her name for the gals in her community is "Sister Goddess."

Sisterhood and the divine feminine play an active role in the Power-Point our leader launches into after a short introduction. I try to take notes in my Pleasure journal. These pages, where I've recorded the effects of my violation, are presently being filled with statistics: on assault, poverty rates for women around the globe, underrepresentation in congress, and the obliteration of female deities. The slides go by too quickly for me to write down numbers, and I'm struggling to connect these data to why I'm here, but then I see the thread: "Pussy."

Mama Gena loves this P-word. I'm more ambivalent. It evokes the crude Brooklynese I grew up with: *My twat is killing me after fucking Vito three times last night.* I wanted a life beyond these base sentences. I imagined myself a refined lady, thanks to all those singing-dancing-acting lessons my mother paid for. But maybe in trying to be cultivated, I ventured too far from essential earthiness.

Slide show still in motion, I start piecing together Mama Gena's gist: if a woman can awaken her Delta of Venus, she'll find a sage between her legs that knows when this femme is hungry, horny, curious, angry, sad, or sated. This pubic triangle can also directly communicate with Venus in the sky—or Isis, Aja, Gaia, and a thousand other goddesses. The best way to reach these divine beings, according to Mama Gena, is through vulva and vagina. In other words, talking to the heavens is best done through lower lips. We even have two sets, so it's a double prayer.

And what about *my* pussy? Or yoni, twat, cunt, pocketbook, beaver, taco, sacred spot, whatever you call her. I've spent so long worrying if she's dysfunctional or victimized. But that's no longer true because of Stephanie. Here in this room, I'm beginning to believe she's a vigorous, untapped reservoir. Can I dip in those waters? How can I dip in those waters?

If I can figure this out, might I be like the women to my right?

Taking up fifteen or so rows is a section containing all the volunteers wearing those nerve-ending T-shirts. They've paired these with sultry costumes: fishnets and combat boots, purple wigs with sparkly tiaras, corsets over jeans, yellow flats, and lots of bras peeking through sheer fabrics. These are the shiniest people I've ever seen. Even though I'm here to discover physical sensation, I suddenly want illumination too. *Are these the same goal?*

As the day continues, I start suspecting, yes. The church of Mama Gena preaches "turn on" within every aspect of our lives. But first, our guru summons the polar opposite. Sitting on the edge of the platform, or down on her stomach propped up on elbows, she elicits stories of lack. Not surprisingly, there are many rape and molestation narratives—but not only. A sixty-something widow in a coifed, gray bob hasn't fooled around in fourteen years; she didn't think this part of her life was important. An eighteen-year-old college student, who could be a Vogue model, despises her breasts. A fifty-two-year-old weight-lifter wed the wrong man, and now she feels trapped. My favorite tale of woe comes from a young Black woman in square, white glasses who says, "So my story is that I'm fucking brilliant. I work in academia. I have a PhD and two master's degrees, y'all. I'm smarter than every one of my colleagues. I'm fucking brilliant and I'm fucking tired of pretending that I'm not."

The crowd explodes in applause. I join them but angst quivers in my gut because this kind of self-assuredness feels foreign, transgressing. Mama Gena says many times, "The patriarchy does not let women play a full set of piano keys." I wonder which keys I play. Isn't it obvious? Being a friction machine, a good daughter who doesn't long for too much, a frightened girl. The keys I'm avoiding? These are less clear.

Mama Gena's activities, interspersed with participant tales of yearning, are meant to unbury these missing keys. Throughout the day, accompanied by dynamic, mood-appropriate music—Bach, Beyonce, Taylor Swift, Miles Davis—we compile a list of one hundred desires; we scream our rage to the heavens, full volume; we confess to a neighbor what we'd like to manifest, while gyrating our hips to stimulate erotic buzz; and so much more.

I love each of these opportunities, but as the day winds down, I'm still searching for a portal to my larger aspiration—rewiring myself for pleasure. I mean, everything we've done has involved desire and delight. But I'm also confused. What should I specifically focus on?

Fostering more anger? Should I put my energy on the desires I wrote on that card? At the top of the list was resurrecting my failed solo play.

Are these circuits related to my sexuality, and am I to reroute these also, one by one?

I'm hoping the closing activity will give me clarification and direction. We are to strut across the stage. It's like this: up the steps house left, shake-your-money-maker, and down the steps house right. Since I'm in the back, and we go row by row, I watch hundreds of attendees let loose, many donning their boas. A few strip down to undergarments. When my turn comes, the DJ switches to Prince, "1999." The vamp is so familiar—*DUM dadadadadum*. I climb the stairs, feeling tired from sharing my pain and yearnings. Also, my wedge boots are too clunky to really let it rip. But then a shift begins.

The stage has always asked more of me than ordinary life. In this rarified space, I immediately unfurl until I'm fully extended. Then, I sync it—body, mind, and artistic vision; graceful limbs, rhythm, and breathing. Even voice is aligned because I'm singing along, not the Prince lyrics but this: *I am sexy.*

Surrendered to the beat, and hundreds of Sister-Goddesses showing their fucking brilliance around me, I'm sexy like a flirty tree. I'm sexy like I was when I danced at Diana and Richard's with my senses hungry-open. I'm sexy like those galaxy-channeling women in the tutus and tiaras and yellow flats. *I am one of these women.* I've always had this ability when I'm under the spotlight. When eyes are watching me. Audience eyes. Male eyes. But I'm not being watched here, not concretely. So this vitality is not about performing. It's about permission.

As I make my way toward the steps, down from the platform, before I leave this expansiveness, I feel the truth vibrating throughout my existence. *I am sexy when I am fully myself. Sexiness is nothing more than fearlessness.*

Back on the ground, in my seat, observing the others, inhaling my boa, I try to grasp it, the pleasure plasticity I came here for—becoming a wildly erotic person. Did it already take effect? Am I forever recircuited?

No.

But Mama Gena was right. I get it now. Full power emerges from an embrace of our complete being. All eighty-eight keys. It makes me think about my bedroom challenges. They've been exclusively focused on terror of men. What if I've always been more afraid of myself?

Out on the street, I rush to meet what's waiting for me outside. No, not a Harley. It's Kurt at a Holiday Inn Express watching CNN. I'm curious how today will affect my functioning. I suppose I'm still searching for the nexus between being sexy and wanting sex.

Alas, even with a little fun from the Holiday Inn mini-bar, I still have low libido and arousal limpness, and orgasm blah. An insight finds its way under these hotel sheets, though: it's not individual wires I need to reconfigure. It's a cohesive set—8,000 nerve endings.

My next stop has to be awakening them.

I think I know how to do it too.

However, going down that path involves the biggest risk of my life.

Tips for *Your* Pleasure Plan

Something to Try:

Take a pleasure day. Map it out in advance, or allow it to proceed spontaneously. Choose nonsexual pleasure activities, so you can explore pleasure without a lot of pressure. Simply choose things you love doing, but do them in aggregate. Here's an example: Go to an afternoon matinee, then browse a fab library, then walk through the park, then stop for a treat that you savor while reading the book you got at the library. Give yourself pleasure after pleasure. Notice how you feel at the end of the day.

P.S. If a full day is not possible, choose an amount of time you can manage. However, still fit in at least two or three pleasure activities.

Journal Prompts:

1. Are there aspects of your day that can be more pleasurable?

   _____

   _____

   _____

2. How might you enhance these parts of your day? Examples include pausing to stretch, dancing for five minutes before the evening news, wearing a favorite item of clothing for no special occasion. . . .

   _____

   _____

   _____

3. If you're resistant to adding more pleasure to your day, why do you think that is?

   _____

   _____

   _____

14

A Tantrika Unshrinks the Vagina

I am on my way to get my clitoris optimized.

I'm trusting my instincts, letting them lead me to nerve endings, even if I've had to use my entire last paycheck for what I'm about to do. It's the Tantrika I phoned when I first began *The Pleasure Plan*. She's the woman who told me I had a shrinking vagina. I need to find out what that is! Also, what else does she know about my package?

When I told Kurt I wanted to see this practitioner, he was not impressed. He was also concerned. A few weeks ago, we attended a workshop together in *Orgasmic Meditation*. There, we watched a live demo of clitoral stimulation that included a woman's exposed vulva, a man's hand, and lots of public moaning. Both of us were very uncomfortable, even triggered.

"This is nothing like that," I told my husband, who came back at me with reservations regarding the Tantrika herself. He reminded me how she initially wanted to see us as a couple, naked.

"She was right," I retorted. "I could have saved years of healing if we'd seen her in the beginning." He didn't disagree. I went on to tell him since I didn't have pain anymore, she could help me solo. I could finally get the erotic awakening I've been seeking. My husband—bless his developing openness—went with my certitude.

A week later, I checked into a boxy corporate hotel in Manhattan, one with a bidet in each room. A bidet—like on my honeymoon. I wanted it as a framing device. Anticipating transformation, I used it to baptize myself just this morning, if you can call a few splashes baptism. Now, bundled up for February New York weather, I'm on my way to see this magic woman.

I'm early, though. I'm never early. Near her apartment, I dash into an Urban Outfitters where I drench myself in honeysuckle cologne. Now I smell like a thirteen-year-old. I layer on a spritzing fragrance with a heavier scent of musk, which isn't more pleasant, but it's mature because I'm not thirteen anymore. Not thirteen at all.

Locating her building a few minutes later, entering the glass and chrome front door of this squat brick apartment complex (circa 1950s), I ride up in a scrubbed elevator. I used to live in a similar building, about a mile from here, so I feel calm, surprisingly, based on what I'm about to do. When I get out of the elevator, there she is, in the doorway. "Are you, Laauwra?" She drags out the syllables of my name in a very charming, Italian way.

"Francesca?"

"Yes! Hi. Come on in."

The first thing I see is a blue leather couch and a massive computer sitting on a desk. We sit and chat about my session, but soon we are moving through the boxcars of her railroad apartment. I follow my hostess as she makes her way into the central hallway. She is as thin and muscular as a dancer. From behind, in her fitted flare dress and gold sandals, along with brown, shiny bob, she has the aura of an ex-showgirl from a bygone era.

"Is it cold out?" she says over her shoulder. The words are ordinary, but her foreign vowels, and retro ambiance, make me feel like we're in a black and white movie, and we are both stars. I'm the anxious one. When we hit the back room, everything becomes Technicolor—with an Eastern flair. Lilac walls, a laminated chakra poster, a blue Chinese scroll. The room could have been decorated by my friend Stacey, the earth mama of my yoga group of friends. Stacey has a gift for making spaces cozy-spiritual. I can almost feel Stacey's hand on my shoulder, a gesture of support. Both my shoulders drop down just imagining this.

Then I notice the bed. A gold comforter covers the expanse of this huge brass surface. It has coordinated pillow shams, complete with tassels. The bed is greedy. It's sucking up the oxygen in this room. My lungs respond with shallow use.

We start seated, though, at the foot of this monster bed. I am settled into a small, round cafe table. Made of white painted wood, it's flanked by two matching Victorian carved chairs that currently contain me and Francesca. She is facing me, almost knee-to-knee, her clingy dress riding slightly up her thighs.

"So, close your eyes," she says, almost in a whisper. "I want you to feel your feet on the ground, feel your grounding. I want you to see how you feel."

How I feel is itchy. I've deliberately worn comfortable clothes—an all-black ensemble of yoga pants, cotton tank, and weathered cardigan. These materials now aggravate my skin. Beneath this epidermal discomfort, my heart thumps wildly.

Soon I am chanting, though.

Francesca wants me to vocalize mantra sounds that are associated with different chakras. These are familiar to me from the yoga world, so I'm glad I can easily follow along—"Lam…Vam…Ram…

Yam…Ham…Om…Om." I intone these seven sounds, over and over. Essentially, we need to make sure each chakra is working—not blocked or too active—before we shift to the next. Francesca is particularly interested in my lowest (Lam) chakra. Near the base of the spine, it oversees feelings of safety. If we don't feel secure, we can't turn on the chakra above, which governs our sensuality.

After about ten minutes of chanting, augmenting alignment and tranquility, Francesca transitions us. "Laura? I'm going to teach you a way of being in your body. It's called *Surrender Breath*." She demonstrates by making little sighs. Then she shapes her mouth, a lovely shade of orange red, into an O. She looks like she is about to whistle, and there *is* a high-pitched sound as she draws in a large amount of air. When she exhales, her eyelids partially close and her bottom lip slackens. A pure, loosened sound emerges from this opening: "Aaaaaaaaaaaaah."

It appears easy to produce. "Ah," I mimic.

"Not Ah. Aaaaaaaaaaaaah. I want you to breathe from the belly, okay?"

"I am."

"No. You're breathing up here." She points to her chest, which is tan, even in the middle of winter. "Do you know how to use the diaphragm?"

Her question grabs my viscera and twists it. I've been an actor for decades. I've been doing diaphragmatic breath work since high school—before! Trying to not sound defensive, I mumble something about theater training and then emphasize my yoga education and practice.

"That's why you're having trouble!" she exclaims. "Yoga has a completely different energy."

I'm confused. Isn't this some kind of yoga?

"Yoga is masculine. It's controlled." She clarifies: She's talking about psychic energies balanced in each individual, not gender identity. "Surrender Breath is the opposite of control," she continues. "It's female energy. It's surrender." Her eyes are shiny when she says this. Even her crow's feet are rays of light—extending all the way to Venus.

"Do you want to try some more before we study the clitoris?"

At that moment a laugh erupts from my gut, exactly the kind of abdominal release she's been coaxing from me for half an hour. Francesca laughs too at this unabashed expression of my anxiety, which takes over my whole being. Involuntarily, I've surrendered to these nerves. This is it. This is Surrender Breath.

"I'd like to know what to expect," I say as I slowly stroll toward the bed. I notice that itchiness again. This time in the crook of an arm, the armpit of the other.

"Sure. This is not like going to be some... some brothel. It's going to be healing."

"I know," I say because it's already healing, despite some lingering itchiness.

"You don't even have to take your clothes off," she says.

Until that moment, I didn't know I had a choice. If I didn't take them off how would she teach me about the 8,000 nerve endings?

"Or I could take off *my* clothes," she offers.

"No! That's okay."

"I just offer because everybody is different. For some people, they feel less... humiliated that way. I will do whatever you need to be safe." There's that safe concept again.

"I want to take my clothes off," I say in a strong, resonant voice, "but only the lower half." Yes, this is what I want.

Without delay, I take everything off from the waist down. Once I'm done and I'm lying on the navy towel she's placed upon the golden comforter, I feel oddly without itch, not jittery. This position is similar to the way I always began vaginal physical therapy. Also, I'm intrigued. Once again I am being attended to—mended—by a post-menopausal woman, like the midwives in my imagination who applied poultices of chamomile, myrrh, and sage.

Francesca presents no herbs, not literally. But if she were alive in those ancient days, I bet she would have used them. In contemporary times, she wants me to continue attempting Surrender Breath. I need more calm before we explore sensations down south. To help, as I "Ahhhhh," the Tantrika places her palms, which are hot, on my abdomen. I've always found warmth in this vicinity soothing, and this is no exception. I'm consciously letting go of tension as Francesca starts moving her hand around my belly in search of a spot she eventually identifies. Located right above my pubic bone, she tells me, there's a little indentation in the flesh. She wants me to feel it with my own hand, but I can't find it, so she suggests switching places.

Without hesitation or sweet talk, she reclines on the happy-color bedspread, putting my hand on her vulva. Well, a tad above, where she leads me to the very top of her mound. "There," she says. With her guidance, I push down right below the swell of her tummy. My hand sinks into a kind of dip. Pleased, she has me tuck my fingers, slightly, behind the upper ridge of her pubic bone.

"See, my muscles here are released, but yours are very tense. Let's release your muscles too."

On my back again, my Tantric teacher, who is crouched over my torso, massages this set of muscles. When I inadvertently sniff her breath, it's pleasant. Always a sign of trustworthiness.

I *do* trust her as she continues her work. Then I watch her hands sink slightly behind my own pubic bone. In that same instant, my genitals unfasten like a reflex—*Open Sesame*. It's like a trigger point, except, instead of sending me into fight or flight or freeze, this touch has the opposite effect: release. It's an *anti*-trigger point.

"You feel that?" she asks with gleaming white teeth.

"I do!" I tell her that even with physical therapy, and its incredible aftermath, this is the first time my genitals have ever fully let go.

"Your yoni is just freaked out," she says.

"It's true! My yoni is freaked out." A satisfying laugh shakes loose a few tears.

Francesca chuckles too. For a few moments, two brunettes on a box spring are talking about all the freaked out yonis in the world. The discussion is cozy, radical in its honesty. Maybe that's why my new guru makes her segue, "Tell me, Laura, how big is your husband's lingam?"

My jaw instantly tightens but this is not about fellatio memories. It's about secrecy. One isn't supposed to talk about such things if one is partnered with a man, who, by nature of being a man, is invested in the world thinking he's well-endowed. I get it: A perception of grandeur is important for a guy's sexual self-esteem. I support that privately. But, according to my jaw, it seems his ego is more important than my own experience, or access to solutions. Because size matters—in ways that have nothing to do with men.

Stephanie asked about Kurt too, during my physical therapy weeks. But this was a technical inquiry related to which dilator I should progress to.

Francesca's investigation goes further. She wants to know if I'm having trouble because my husband is on the large side. I emphasize that my troubles began when I was thirteen, with tampons, so size has never been the source of my problems. Yet, undeniably, phallus dimensions have determined how penetration plays out.

I tell the Tantrika about a guy I dated in grad school. He was one of the three beaus I was extremely attracted to before I met Kurt. Prior to getting naked the first time, this fellow grad school student warned me he had a huge penis and that a lot of women couldn't take it. Deeply infatuated, I wanted to prove I wasn't a pussy with a tiny pussy. But that's exactly what I was. Every time we got physical, I bled. When I confided to a couple of friends, they were empathic but had no advice. A buddy told me she bled too during lovemaking, on occasion. Reluctantly, I saw a gynecologist, who told me nothing was wrong except this fellow was too much for me. My man eventually ended our relationship, saying he didn't think he could ever fall in love with me.

Francesca is here for guidance around these matters, the first I've ever had. She informs me that though Kurt is not quite as large as this "boy in school," I still need full arousal before penetration. Otherwise, the opening to the vagina, which she calls the introitus, will freak out as it's used to. She's right. The dilators made intercourse more comfortable, yet entering is still sometimes painful.

Now that we've cleared that up, it's time to advance to what I came here for. My teacher suggests it: "I want you to know how to pleasure yourself with the clitoris."

Then she says, "So, do you know where the clitoris is, I mean on your body?"

I leap at this opportunity to show off. It's taken me three years to reach this apex of knowledge. "It's right here," I say, lying back down and grazing the delicate area where my inner labia meet.

Francesca plops down beside me. "Yes, that's it," she says, peering in. "But you need to lift up the hood."

"I've already done that."

"No, you haven't."

"Isn't this the clit?" I ask, indicating the tip of wrinkled skin I am holding between pointer and thumb.

"That's still only the hood."

"Really?" *How could I not know this is still only the hood?* "Do you mind if I touch you?" Francesca asks. When I nod, she generates heat, rubbing her palms together. That heat transfers to my privates. "So you pull this up, okay? . . . *Here* is the clitoris. Of course, when you're aroused, it will be much bigger."

I have to strain my neck to see, but there is a shiny head slyly poking through a modest hole.

"I didn't know," I say, feeling the electrons from her hands, somehow, transferring to my eye sockets. Warm tears might flow.

"That's why you're here," she says with a compassionate laugh. "Do you know how few women know their clitoris is like that?"

I want to believe her, but I feel like an idiot. After thirty years of screwing, after three solid years of sexological research, how could I not identify my clit? "Do you have a mirror?" I ask.

"Yes. But that's not the whole clitoris."

What?

She starts telling me about the internal clitoris. I suddenly recall Diana talking about it too, at her retreat. At that event, my yoni was so overwrought I couldn't properly listen. Francesca is setting me straight. The clitoral button (glans) extends down on both sides, running underneath the inner labia, about 3 or 4 inches. "It makes a wishbone shape," she states. Then she gets the mirror.

Like Lewis and Clark in lipstick, the Tantric mistress and I explore my territory. I trace the inner clitoris, now that I know where it is.

I also learn my little love button is far away from the vaginal opening. The closer it is, apparently, the easier it is to climax during inter-course—no wonder I have such trouble in this department.

"You probably need to stimulate yourself during intercourse to have an orgasm," Francesca advises.

Where else was I ever going to get this information?

She continues, "When a woman is turned on, the clitoris, both internal and external, fires up. You get, you know, lubrication and blood. This is engorgement. But a woman doesn't stay engorged. She needs to continue arousal throughout."

This explains my experience! Arousal has never felt stable to me, like how it's described by Masters and Johnson, whom I read when I first started my recovery project. Their model for female sexual response is excitement, plateau, orgasm, resolution. In other words, excitement reliably climbs higher and higher. It's not like that for me. My turn-on spikes and drops throughout lovemaking.

A book I recently read, *Come as You Are*, is more consistent with what the Tantrika is saying. But I'm only now connecting the dots. That author, Emily Nagoski, a well-esteemed sex educator, says a woman's sexual response is comprised of a brake pedal and an accel-erator. All aspects of making love—from the decision to engage, to the acts themselves, to the emotions afterward—are related to those pedals. A good place to start discovering our sensual selves, the author advises, is to investigate what deactivates *No*, and what activates *Go*.

Which leads me to this: *Can I release my brake enough for Francesca to stroke me too? Might I discover, in this room, my yoni's potential for fun?*

After I grant permission, Francesca lays her hand back on my stomach, having me do the "Ahs" of Surrender Breath, to ground me.

Soon the flat pads of her fingers are tracing a path up and down my clitoral hood, barely brushing against it. As I continue respiration (almost steady), she narrates what she's doing. Most activity is on the upper right-hand quadrant of my clitoral glans—what she calls "the one o'clock position." She clarifies that this locale is from the perspective of a person glancing at the vulva. Apparently, there's a standard clit-clock.

But let's talk about sensation. What's going on, because of her expert touch, is "engorgement"…followed by gradual moisture.…But now my *non*-clitoral head tells me that I don't want to climax here. What I want is a pause.

As Francesca goes to get me water, I glance around this tapestry-rich, Eastern-flair lair, feeling like I've been here for days. My ninety-minute session must be completely over, no? If that's the case, it's fine. I've definitely gotten the brass ring I was hoping to grab.

When she returns, sitting on the bed with me, the Tantrika informs me that tantra is so much more than knowing about our bits. Its lofty aims involve awakening our consciousness so we might discover profound communion with life itself and that which provides its force—God, Goddess, the Universe, Tao, whatever you name it. Listening to her, I'm reminded of why I initially called this woman, back when she happened to be driving down that mountain. I still want all that divine union. But, first, I need to build a better foundation of basic sex ed.

And that's exactly what Francesca is suggesting, in an expanded form. "So one more thing I'm offering now," she says, patting my leg for comfort. "If you want, I can go inside and do your G-spot."

Every sinew in my body is fatigued like I have Spanish Fly flu, so I'm unsure. Francesca speaks to my tiredness, "You know, it takes a lot of energy to do this exploration. But you also *get* a lot of energy—from Eros. That's why most people don't even know I'm seventy-two."

This seems utterly impossible.

"I'll show you my driver's license," she says, turning her fit body as if she might fetch it.

"That's all right. I trust you." Maybe sex is not the true elixir. It's *Yes*—the accelerator pedal for all our desires and dreams.

"Let's do it," I say. Then I assume the position (knees open, feet together) as she pours a puddle of coconut oil into her hand, her lubricant of choice.

"Aaaaaaaaaah," Francesca intones, wanting me to repeat after her as she enters me. There's tightness at first, but not much.

I'm just inside," she says "And now…I'm at the G-spot."

"Really?" I say because what she's touching doesn't feel age-reversing in the least. I just need to pee. She tells me this is normal. Lots of women have this experience when this area, which she also calls the "urethral sponge," is touched. She assures me this sensation often goes away when a woman becomes more aroused.

I take her word for it as she shows me how to reach this spot myself.

With Francesca's coaching, I curve my index finger in a "come here" gesture so I can access the mysterious locale. The texture is ridged, or lined…like lines of Braille. This image seems apt. I am learning to read myself.

For the rest of this activity, and the remainder of the session, which ends shortly afterward, I keep coming back to this Braille metaphor. As I leave Francesca's, thanking her, I'm ready to open this book in private.

When I get back to my bidet hotel, what I experience—that night and the next morning, several times—is healing. But it's my own hands. My hands have the ability to provide safety, surrender, anxiety relief, brake release, titillation, stimulation, engorgement, more accelerator pedal, re-engorgement, and hair-to-toenail pleasure—in no set order.

I am my own healer. I suppose it's always been this way. I just didn't know.

Zoom.

I can't believe it.

Zoom.

Tips for *Your* Pleasure Plan

Something to Try:

Explore your body while alone (the tub or shower is fine if you can't find time to lie in bed). Find places on the body that, when touched, relax the whole nervous system. Keep going until you find these areas. You may be surprised where they are.

Journal Prompts:

1. Is there any place in the world where you feel completely safe?

   _____

   _____

   _____

2. If you don't feel safe anywhere, what relaxes you? Write about anything that calms or soothes you.

   _____

   _____

   _____

3. Do you know your genital anatomy? (See the Recommended Resource section in the Appendix for info.)

   _____

   _____

   _____

4. Can you distinguish between feeling uncomfortable and feeling unsafe? If you're interested in moving beyond a lot of *No*, can you explore your comfort edge within a greater context of feeling safe?

   _____

   _____

   _____

15

Fearless Flying

I'm high in the sky, 30,000 feet. Kurt and I are on a plane making its way to Indiana, where I've been offered opportunities so strange and exhilarating I have trouble accepting they're real. It makes me think about a sentence my guy has been uttering lately: "It's like you're someone else." He's talking about my constant enthusiasm for carnality. Eight months after seeing the Tantrika, my libido has stayed as elevated as this jet.

Take last Thursday.

At around six, Kurt arrived home with take-out because I'd requested that our intimacy predominantly transpire before 8:00 PM *and* that it be unhooked from chopping, sautéing, marinating, stewing, and crusty dishes. I know lots of folks find cooking sensual, but given my circumstances—wee kitchen, lack of dishwasher, and a personal energy level in the evening hovering around zero—I do not. And guess what? Rather than being blindsided by a horny hubby in moonglow, I found I could ask for romance when the sun is still out. Talk about leaving the lights on! But let us not overlook a salient detail: *I was the one doing the asking.*

After dinner, we adjourned to the bedroom where wantonness poured out of me: "Do you think you can massage my back and legs?" It was followed by another request: "Don't touch my genitals, Babe, not until I say so—*if* I say so—because I might want to stroke myself." Being able to enjoy erotic contact without pressure has been a magic formula for me these past eight months. *I'm loving the constant tease.* And then there is the variety. I was right to suspect novelty's prominence when it comes to my arousal. But I'm no longer afraid it will lead me astray like I was at Diana and Richard's workshop. From role play to costumes to cut-up fruit—yes, tons of cantaloupe—I get what I need, as long as I'm vocal. I can't believe it's taken me thirty-plus years to have a voice.

I'm not saying there aren't additional landscapes to explore. There are. For instance, I'm still figuring out direct clitoral stimulation, why it's mostly too intense, and I do *not* fancy G-spot pressure (yet?). But I *am* enjoying hard cock inside me now. How's that for transmutation? I even have my next adventure mapped out.

And speaking of travel, at our current speed of 500 miles per hour, Kurt sits to my right, at the window. To my left, on the aisle, is a middle-aged lady who scowled at me when I accidentally used her seat belt thirty minutes ago. I've let this go because of where we're headed—Indiana University. I've been invited to conduct a workshop on sexual assault prevention *and* give a talk on resilience. The latter includes excerpts from my play, which unbelievably, has been resurrected (with major edits). Recently, I placed it in two Fringe Festivals as well as another festival Off-Broadway. And a few months ago, an essay based on the same material was published in the *New York Times*. The freakin' *New York Times*. It's not solely my love life that's been transformed. It's my whole career, my entire life.

I trace a lot of this back to Francesca. At that visit, when we talked about the strength of one chakra being the foundation for the next, we concentrated mostly on the first chakra, governing safety, as well as the second, which oversees sexual vitality. Well, guess what sits above? Power. Chakra Three, located in the solar plexus, or *kishkas* as my mother would say, is all about different manifestations of power. I feel the triumvirate of One, Two, and Three working now in my airplane seat as I look out Kurt's window feeling stable and juicy and courageous and happy.

But now I have to pee.

If I'm honest, I'll admit it: I've had to urinate for fifteen minutes, maybe more. I've held it in because I was busy with my energy-wheel superpowers. Also, there's that female on my left. She already admonished me once, facially at least, regarding the buckle mishap. It's my own fault I'm in this pickle, anyway. They've already served us drinks. I should have excused myself as soon as the cart started clanging from the back galley. I had a slight urge then, didn't I?

I glance at my elimination obstacle. While sipping a ginger ale, she's reading a novel using black-framed readers. Her fingers are covered in dented silver rings, the kind I've seen at contemporary art museums. In her jeans and blazer, she resembles my friend's mother, an interior designer. There is no way I'm going to bother her.

But whoa there. This is the old me talking. I am no longer a mini, compressed woman. Didn't my husband confirm my alteration just last Thursday? I swivel my bod toward him, my numero uno fan. "Can I put this here?" I ask, indicating my cup of sparkling water and my empty bag of pretzels.

"Sure." He launches into helpful hubby mode, transferring my debris to his table. I'm hoping this voluminous activity will inspire the traveler on my left to rise so I don't need to ask her. She remains absorbed in her book.

So I unclasp my seat belt with as much extra movement as I can get away with. I'm practically getting up to stretch.

She doesn't seem to notice. As a writer, can I begrudge her loving a good book? Of course not. Be that as it may, my situation is getting critical.

"Excuse me," I say.

As she faces me, I see challenge in her brown eyes. She doesn't say anything—or get up. Anger seeps into my jawline like heavy sand weighing down my gums. Words stumble out anyway, "I'm sorry. I hate to disturb you." I point to the lavatory behind us.

After a loud sigh, she becomes a pantomime artist. Her gestures are that exaggerated. A larger-than-life version of a person who must put down a book and fold a tray table and locate a spot on the floor for her two drinks, so they won't topple. It's tricky; I'll give her that.

During her performance, I catch a glimpse of Kurt. With bared teeth, his eyebrows are almost up to the luggage bin, as in *Yikes!* I'm relieved. It's not just me: this woman is scary. But who does she think she is? Finally, she stands, theatrically, allowing me to pass.

As I shimmy out and walk up the aisle, my jaw is no longer dragging. It pulsates with blood that's churned upstairs by those lower chakra wheels. Once I'm in the lavatory, I'm pissed, even after I fully piss. Then I gaze into the mirror. The blue light of the 737's bathroom illuminates my reflection, along with a strange thought—*I'm not afraid of her*. These words slosh around my system, until I feel their racing effect, like three cups of espresso. Heart beating hard, I ask myself: *Have I always been afraid of rude people?* I have to answer *Yes*. Rudeness is a form of abuse, and, too often, I've taken it in stride, as if abuse were normal. It's not. I point at my image in the mirror as if it's her, that mean lady. She's right here with me. Then I start to giggle.

It's the setting: the site of the eight-mile-high club. Every adult book I stole a glimpse of in the 1970s—when I was too young to be absorbing such things—featured people fucking in airplane restrooms. I think of the stack of dirty novels I found in my father's room when I was twelve. In one of them, Erica Jong's *Fear of Flying*, there's no jet screwing, per se, but air travel *is* used as a metaphor for female desire. Jong immortalized the phrase *zipless fuck*. She inspires me now to declare, *I don't give a fuck*. In other words—I need to scold my seating companion, for real. I have to let her know she has transgressed, and I will not tolerate this behavior.

Other people must be waiting to use the restroom, so I have to psyche myself into this, quickly. *What if she yells at me? What if she tells the crew I'm a terrible person with an abnormal bladder? Shhhhhh,* I whisper to my neuroses. I conjure all the ways I've been opening my mouth these days—without worrying what people think. Every instance has contributed to my altered state. In the sci-fi blue light, I concentrate on a dinner party a few months ago.

We had run into one of Kurt's colleagues in the packed living room. After my husband introduced him and his role in the office, this Swiss gentleman, who was wearing a suit and tie at this relaxed event, asked about my own profession. I told him I was a playwright.

"How fabulous," he said with a clap. "Do you write on any particular topics?"

I told him I was reworking a play about healing from childhood sexual abuse. It came out matter-of-factly, which surprised me. Sharing the topic of my work was terrifying when I first started *The Pleasure Plan*, but I guess I had gotten used to these conversations. Speaking casually that night about how abuse had affected me made me feel like I'd crossed over a shame line.

"So your drama is about trauma," said the Swiss man after hearing more about my play. He seemed pleased with his rhyming phrase. Then his face changed. "Trauma is an interesting topic," he told me. "My wife…Kurt knows this…but my wife died eight months ago, of an aneurism." He put a hand on his chest.

For the next five minutes, while people around us chatted about work or Netflix or merlot, he revealed his struggles raising three children without a mother. This foreigner was so formal and reserved, yet liquid emotion poised at the corner of his eyes. He let it be there, and I joined him with sadness in my own corners. Though our talk was heavy, there was liberation between us. Communion.

Subsequent to that dinner party, and especially after resurrecting my play, I've been having frequent exchanges like this. A woman recently told me her brother was schizophrenic. Others have disclosed they too have been victimized by pedophiles—most of these confessors have been men. In every instance, I'd found connection by refusing to be intimidated by what I'm pursuing, by who I am.

I refuse to be intimidated.

That's what I say to myself as I march back to my seat. A motor in my belly (Chakra Three?) seems revved. When I get to my row, shockingly, the interior designer gets right up. But once I've entered and settled, the show again commences. Sighing, she puts her tray table down, moves her beverages from the floor, and places them back on her tray. Soon enough, we're situated. The moment has passed. The thing is, I need this verbalization to prove that I've shifted, permanently. How do I get her to confirm my new identity?

The words drop onto my dome and seep in. I stare at her as it comes out—the most forceful phrase I've uttered in fifty-one years on this planet: "I'm sorry, but I had to pee."

She returns my stare. Her eyes appear clear like they once had cataracts but no longer. Perhaps she sees I am worthy of respect. Even if she doesn't, I see it in her eyes, even when she turns them back to her book.

Leaning my head back, stretching out my legs, drinking my fizzy drink again, I start reading too, the in-flight magazine. I stumble upon an ad for Hong Kong. People in a rooftop restaurant are dining and thrilled. Stars above hint at greater galaxies.

So much is beyond this day of travel. After my workshop and talk, I'll enter the next phase of my quest—a masturbation weekend, a whole seminar. I tip my hat to the person I have become. But it's time to experience massive, consistent, multiple, ecstatic orgasms.

Maybe I'll find that I am becoming and becoming.

Tips for *Your* Pleasure Plan

Something to Try:

What's something scary that you want? Can you ask for it? If you can't, or you think it's simply not possible to have it, ask a person you deem knowledgeable, or simply someone in your corner, how you might go about turning your desire into reality.

Journal Prompts:

1. Is there something you need to say to someone but you're too afraid?

   _____

   _____

   _____

2. What are you afraid might happen if you speak up?

   _____

   _____

   _____

3. What might happen if you don't speak up?

   _____

   _____

   _____

16

How to Have an Orgasm, or Two, or Three

A
nd now, the final frontier.

"Get naked," says the fleshy woman with spiked blond hair, who has just let me into her apartment. "Disrobe and enter the temple." Her raspy voice reminds me of how much women smoked in the seventies, especially liberated icons like the one standing before me. She looks to be sixty-six. She's not. She's eighty-six. This is Betty Dodson, a sexologist who invented Second Wave Feminism, along with Gloria Steinem and others. Betty's piece of the emancipation puzzle was teaching women to maximally have pleasure. To that end, she developed a masturbation technique I'm here to uncover. I've come too far to not know how to come very far.

Betty points out hooks upon which I'm to hang up my clothes. Then she sashays away. I begin undressing with a thumping in my torso. A two-day workshop in the buff is scary, for sure. Just as nerve-wracking is disclosing how much I don't know about ecstasy—despite years of research. So many questions. *Why am I able to climax by myself but not with a lover? Are those little waves during lovemaking, the ones that recently started, considered orgasm? Should climax be earth-shattering? If so, what am I doing wrong?* A residual cloak of shame has kept me from getting these answers. But now that I'm discarding layers, education awaits.

Nude, I enter the temple.

Or, if you prefer, Betty's immaculate living room in Midtown Manhattan. The sacred and stylish coexist here. A plush, slate-gray carpet touches walls decorated with drawings and paintings; Betty is also an artist. In many of these works, women are in sensual repose. The real thing is strikingly more present. Three bare-naked ladies are sitting on the floor in BackJack chairs. These places are arranged in a circle, at the center of which is a silver tray with lighted candles. That's our altar.

"Hi, I'm Laura," I say, taking an empty seat and crossing my ankles so I'm not completely exposed.

"I'm Desiree," smiles a young woman to my left with a flat tummy and a flower tattoo on her left shoulder.

I try not to notice her pubic grooming choice but do anyway (her legs are not very crossed). She's got a wide landing strip, like me. I'm curious how many of us waxed for this occasion.

"Where are you traveling from?" asks Desiree. She goes on to tell me she's from Ohio. The woman across from us, closer to my age, with magenta hair down to the middle of her back, hails from Vancouver. Before we get further into our chat, more women arrive, until we are complete. Eight people with unveiled vulvas and breasts.

Then Betty comes in with Carlin, her business partner. Carlin is statuesque with long, blond hair and a smile that's tremendous and generous. She's very quick to laugh. A former lawyer, she quit her job so she could dedicate her life to preserving Betty's legacy. Betty is just as striking but gruffer. Hailing from the Midwest, with a PhD in sexology, she's got the spirit of cabbies, sanitation workers, and postal employees (my dad included) who populated the neighborhood where I grew up. It's a particular down-to-earth quality that contrasts, and complements, her academic creds. An example of her vibe is what she says next: "What we're going to do now is tell our history of fucking, or fucking history," she informs. "We need to know what has gotten in the way of your pleasure, so we can get rid of it. Don't worry how long your story takes. Take the time you need! And tell me EVERYTHING. I'm a Virgo. I like details! You dig?"

"Yup," I say along with others. And the tales begin. I go early on, elucidating my project, which I feel proud of. I unhook my ankles, occasionally, because it's okay to be seen here. Every one of us has a complicated history. The woman with pink hair, a fellow New Yorker, was preyed upon as a teen; a nurse from New Zealand just discovered she's bisexual; a Columbian architect has never had satisfying intimacy with her husband. I'm tuned in to these woes and discoveries. I love being part of this tribe. However, underneath, almost imperceptibly, I am comparing myself. I am comparing my body.

It's subtle but pernicious. It's also confusing. I've spent decades accepting my physical form, after tons of adolescent teasing. The worst culprit was Sarah, my childhood neighbor, who told me for years that my ears stuck out like Dumbo's, my chest was flat, and my nose was identical to a witch on a Saturday morning TV show. There was also judgment of my toes, tush, stomach, skin... well, all of me.

I already felt awkward around boys because of being abused. Sarah's take on my attractiveness compounded a suspicion I was unlovable. It's one of the reasons I dated, almost exclusively, men with whom I had no chemistry—until I met Kurt. After we met, he made a point of telling me every day how beautiful I was until I began believing him. He continues this tradition, but I no longer doubt him. Or I thought that was the case.

Sitting in this living room with other yearning females, I'm not sure why these old insecurities have arisen. I'm curious if they're connected to another person in the room—Betty herself. At eighty-six, she's youthful and vibrant. She also happens to be built like my mother. It's been many years since I've seen my mother, let alone without clothes. I'd forgotten what she looked like, but here she is, in a way. Via Dr. Dodson, I'm viewing Mom's perfect proportions, her strong arms and thighs, her pendulous-but-firm breasts, her soft belly. I speculate that seeing Betty brings up ancient shame. My mom's relationship with her body was not ideal. Don't I pat my own soft belly, often, obsessed that I too am getting fat? As Betty describes our next activity, I'm excited to transform any body issues tenaciously hanging out.

So what if ridding my shame entails showing this crowd my clitoris?

The exercise is called Show and Tell, and it's something Dodson has been doing since Jimmy Carter was president. She began these Bodysex workshops because too many colleagues and friends believed their vulvas were ugly or deformed, not having seen others', except for girly magazines. She had the same unease about her own attractiveness down there. But what if she could reveal to women our real, gorgeous array? Forty years after initiating these sessions, she's only found an increased need for her work, given the prevalence of porn. Our sassy octogenarian says finding fault with our bodies—from our ears (thanks, childhood friend Sarah) to our labia—is a major barrier to lust and satisfaction.

Yay to getting rid of barriers.

Here's how Show and Tell works. One by one, we sit next to Betty as the group scoots in close to examine our goods. Then Betty gives each vulva a name, while Carlin snaps a picture that she sends by email. We only get photos of ourselves! I suppose that's why no one present at the workshop expresses worry these images will end up in the wrong internet hands. We trust the integrity of this community. Before we begin the live reveal, Betty and Carlin show us videos and drawings of genital anatomy—internal and external. These materials celebrate our sexual biodiversity, which is exactly what I encounter via the seven other participants, as I scoot in close to their coochies. I see lips shaped like wings, petals, ears, shells, or just themselves. Inner labia are longer than outer labia, and vice versa. Some gals have no labia at all. Pussies are blush, mocha, mahogany, scarlet, mauve, or tan. Most are a mixture of colors. And then there are the clits and their little heads. I see clitoral glans hidden under hoods (like mine), glans poking out, and glans with no hood. Not a single person in this room has symmetry. I strangely do not measure myself to what I'm witnessing. I'm too fascinated. But, also, we haven't yet gotten to my vaj.

As my turn approaches, I'm sure they'll find me lovely—or not. I run to the bathroom to splash. *What if I smell?* It's irrational. I don't have an infection. I rarely get them. Unless there's an infection—I learned years ago, somehow—a woman should not have an unpleasant odor emanating from her alcove. But I grew up in a house where my mom frequently used douches, another of her body quirks. She advised me to do the same once I hit my teens, and I listened. Only when I moved out, after college, did I discover I didn't need these practices or products. The vagina cleans itself. That said, someone at the workshop mentioned earlier that it's a good idea to pull back the hood in the shower, getting water on the glans itself. Apparently, women also get smegma.

I hope that's not the case with me. Because, now, I'm the vulnerable gal sitting next to our teacher in the designated BackJack chair. Betty angles the makeup mirror and lamp so I can view myself, and others can better investigate my privates. The heat from the light makes me feel like I'm sunbathing nude with my legs open. My bottom sweats into the fabric of the chair.

"Let's see what we have here," Betty states. My sisters adjust their glasses, point, and smile. Then our teacher identifies structures highlighted in her instructional videos and drawings. These are the same bits I explored with Francesca, and to some extent Stephanie, my PT. To tell you the truth, because of my complications, I haven't studied myself very much over the years. What I discover today is that there's less pink than I remember, and more gray hair. However, Betty's maternal hand is around my shoulder, and her temperature is hot—still hot after all these years. After Carlin snaps a picture, Betty names me Dusky Rose.

Ms. Dobson thinks a positive body image starts with adoring our love parts. Self-love emanates from this relationship.

So does orgasm.

That's the focus of tomorrow—why I'm here. Dusky Rose and I don't want anything standing in the way.

The following day as I go back into the living room, taking the same seat, I notice an addition to my left. Next to each chair is now a round silver tray similar to the altar in the center of the room. On each of these surfaces are a bottle of almond oil, a box of tissues, a cordless Magic Wand vibrator (think back massager from the eighties), a condom, and a rectangular box containing a metal rod known as a

Barbell. Betty and Carlin in the buff—everyone is naked again on day two—tell us about this stainless-steel tool. About six inches long and two inches in diameter in the center, the metal is shaped with balls at both ends, one larger than the other. Technically, this is a pelvic floor exerciser, but Betty, working with a medical supply company, had this device augmented for her purposes.

As we attendees touch our toys, nervously anticipating later this afternoon when we'll use them to masturbate en masse, our hostesses tell us why we have this combination of technology. We need them for our erections.

Not male hard-ons, but our own.

I covered some of this terrain with the Tantrika, but now Betty goes further into tumescence. Apparently, women have even more erectile tissue than men, or just as much, if you take into account our collection of swelling areas: the clitoris (including head, hood, shaft, and legs); vestibular bulbs that hug the opening of the vagina; the G-spot, which is actually a sponge surrounding the whole urethra; and another swelling area at the bottom of the vagina, above the perineum, known as the perineal sponge. And that's just a genital hard-on. Nipples get hard too, of course. Also, our ears! According to our guru goddesses, a person with a vulva and/or vagina will have a much better experience when all these areas, or most of them, swell with blood. In fact, Betty says females need twenty to thirty minutes of stimulation in order to have maximum pleasure and orgasm.

In a flash, for the first time, I understand why I can't climax with Kurt—or any man before him. I've only been getting chubbies. A chubby is what my husband calls a partial erection. Betty's technique is specifically designed to circumvent chubbies, by covering more landscape.

But there's more. Taking a break to eat chocolate chip cookies in Betty's sparkling-clean galley kitchen, massaging my sinuses to help my brain absorb everything I've learned so far, I discover the newest trend in sexology: *Responsive Desire*. This means that a hunger for sexual activity, horniness, is now thought to emerge from arousal. Turn-on is first.

This idea is even reflected in the updated version of the *DSM*, where, at the very beginning of *The Pleasure Plan*, I went to diagnose myself. At that time, low desire—or Hypoactive Sexual Desire Disorder (HSDD)—was a thing. But it's disappeared in this updated manual. Or rather, it's been replaced with another designation, Female Sexual Interest-Arousal Disorder (FSIAD). The twenty-first century should be the century of the female hard-on.

Maybe it already is. Case in point, it's time for our circle jerk.

Betty calls her technique Rock 'n' Roll, and that's the music she puts on to serenade us—Jimmy Hendrix to be precise. We've already been instructed what to do, and so we begin. I rub the oil on my vulva to start arousal and to lubricate. Then, we place our individual vibrator on choice parts (with a condom on the dome since these are not for keeps). Next, I grease up the Barbell and begin penetration, using the prescribed rocking motion of the hips—moving the pelvis forward while squeezing PC muscles, then relaxing these muscles as the pelvis swings back.

Each yoni in the room is doing the same. Is it weird? You betcha! But there's also something primal about it, just like in a book I've been reading, *Sex at Dawn*. In this beautifully researched tome, the authors argue that the mating habits of humans directly spring from bonobos, one of the primates we supposedly evolved from. Bonobo culture is exquisitely nonviolent. Part of the reason for this is the way females ease tensions by rubbing their clitorises against each other, a behavior known as Genital-Genital (or GG) rubbing.

I wouldn't dream of pressing against any of these tribe ladies as they experiment with Betty's technique. Mostly, eyes around the room are closed, for privacy. Mine too. But not to surrender. I'm more fascinated than physically excited. In other words, my brain is what's engorged here. But that's okay. I want to record what's going on, like when I started the Screw Journal, which morphed into *The Pleasure Plan* journal. Being in my head like this means I, surely, do not climax. Instead, thankfulness (for this information) spreads throughout my body. It's a different kind of wave, but also one of ecstasy.

After we're done experimenting, we have a long chat about orgasms. It turns out many women in the group are sexperts themselves. They offer their own understanding of orgasm. Apparently, tantra makes a distinction between orgasm and climax. The latter is going over the edge, a full release. But the former is waves of pleasure throughout—exactly what I experience with my lover.

In other words, I'm already having partnered orgasms! They began once my pain subsided. I just didn't know this was real or normal. Betty tells us about a technique for maximizing these small contractions. She calls it edging: as a woman presses close to orgasm, she pulls back, over and over. In this way the waves build and crash into each other, creating their own kind of rapture.

As I bid farewell to these amazing experiential sex researchers, I reflect upon the real legacy of Betty Dodson—females, or those with female parts, talking to each other about what we know, passing down wisdom that contradicts misinformation coming from pornography and media, even doctors.

My intellect is exhausted when I leave Betty Dodson's apartment, but my skin is tingly. I'm anxious to try this fun with my husband.

✳

Fresh from Betty's workshop, I make my way to the country. Kurt and I are spending a few days with Wendy and her husband, who've arranged a guest cottage just for me and my love, a large converted toolshed everyone calls the Love Shack.

Once my husband and I are alone on the foldout bed, after dinner with our friends, I take out the metal rod (we got to keep these), as well as a purple vibrator I bought before trekking upstate, plus a bottle of coconut oil. Then I replicate what I did at the workshop. I'm trying to rub erectile areas, while using the rod and also the phallic-shaped vibrator. It gets complicated. The real obstacle, however, is patience. It's taking a long time for me to get more than a chubby. I keep saying to myself: *That's fine. It's enough. Let's get to the real action.*

But what *is* the real action?

Intercourse?

Someone mentioned foreplay at the workshop, but it didn't register until now. If what I'm doing is a warm-up act for fucking, that's false. Maybe our entire concept of sex is wrong then—femme arousal is not foreplay, it's not fore' anything. It's its own thing. It's pleasure.

So, in other words, there's no need to rush here, right?

And that's when it happens for me, gradually. Using all my gadgets and techniques, taking my expansion seriously, I have a peak orgasm, just like I do on my own. Then, during intercourse—which, I decided, is optional just like any other sensual activity—I experience little waves. But by using edging, they're more connected to each other and rhythmic with my mate.

Kurt and I are instruments playing their own arrangement of the same score. We meld, harmonically. Two people. Three orgasms. Not simultaneous—far apart, in fact—but close enough to sound great. To be great.

To finally, unbelievably, be great.

Tips for *Your* Pleasure Plan

Something to Try:

See Recommended Resources section in the Appendix for illustrations of the female anatomy.

And check out Betty's website for all kinds of wonderful sex education, *https://dodsonandross.com/*.

Journal Prompts:

1. What sensory stimulation might be added to your repertoire to expand your arousal/erection? Visual delights? A taste sensation? Music? Something touching your skin? Scents?

   _____

   _____

   _____

2. Would you like to explore kink or fetish play? See Recommended Resources section in the Appendix.

   _____

   _____

   _____

3. Do you need other sources of fantasy, erotica, and/or porn? See Recommended Resources section in the Appendix.

   _____

   _____

   _____

Journal Prompts (continued):

4. When you're with a partner, do you transition into intercourse/penetration before you're fully aroused? If so, what could you say to a partner in order to give yourself the time and attention you need—and deserve?

   _____

   _____

   _____

5. If arousal is an issue for medical or other reasons, what could you say to your partner that would invite innovative solutions that allow you both to still have intimacy?

   _____

   _____

   _____

17

The Pain Specialist

The pain is back.

It returns several months after Betty Dodson. Kurt and I are making love in the afternoon. We've put blankets on the floor in front of our bed, our room darkened by a rainstorm. The ambiance is soulfully romantic, just like the last months of amazing *unioning*. But soon into our intimate dance, my vajayjay starts stinging—and he's only going down on me. Stinging has *never* been present during this act. When we get to penetration, the burning is worse than ever. It's like my vulva and vagina have come down with a pernicious rash. But this is no skin ailment. It's vestibulitis, the nerve condition physical therapy supposedly cured.

I switch positions, going on the bottom. My mind is on the ceiling, though, as I try figuring out *Why has my problem recurred?* I flash to the plethora of PT maintenance I've been doing: daily Kegels and monthly dilators, plus penetration once or twice a week. Yet, angry neurons assault, and my muscles clamp down, just like in the old days. *Get Out!* they say to my husband's penis, using their own language of tightness and blocking. *Get off me.*

I don't stop, however, because I need to provide friction. It's an ancient way of handling this fiasco, I know. I'm too blindsided to find a better way. I paste on a smile for the duration—until he comes.

The next time my husband and I make love, the snag is just as bad, but I'm vocal at least.

"Go slow. Go slow. Go slow," I say with my eyes pressed closed.

"It hurts?"

"Yeah."

"Shit!"

"I need to stop," I say after a few minutes more, pulling my yoni away from her mate.

"Of course," Kurt responds, helping me uncouple. "You think it's vaginismus?" he asks once we're lying on our sides, married face to married face.

"I think so," I say with heavy sighs that continue for some time. Although, I also manage to give Kurt a blow job. I guess I'm a fellatio multitasker.

The next time Kurt and I meet up for an appointed rendezvous, a few days later, I bow out due to bloating. The instance after that, I'm exhausted. I start sinking into a tar pit of perplexity: *Is this trauma resurfacing? Am I afraid of finally having what I always wanted? Do I have another medical issue I'm not aware of?*

The way I reach Dr. Williams is through a vagina that's not my own. Specifically, it's a book I chance upon at the library. An anonymous author describes her own sexual healing odyssey, which was aided by a gynecologist specializing in pelvic pain. Reading this memoir, my head grows as veiny-pink as my irritated membranes. How could I do my *Oy-My-Vagina-Hurts* project for *five years* and not understand there are doctors whose expertise is achy penetration. Perhaps if I'd grown up trusting the medical community, I would have sought this help sooner. I cut myself some slack here and undertake a mission—to find one of these doctors.

I discover one in New York. Yup, back I go to my ancestral home. This time, I'm in prime real estate, the Manhattan neighborhood of SoHo with its designer shops and trust-fund-hipster restaurants. Three blocks from the building where this doctor's suite resides, I notice something sweeter, an Italian lingerie store. Not Intimissimi. This retail heaven, La Perla, makes some of the most exquisite, and exorbitant, little nothings in the world. I vow to peruse this shop right after my appointment.

First, I have a date with a speculum. A pricey one.

The chance to see this expert is a whopping 1,200 dollars, and, naturally, they don't take insurance. I'm extremely lucky Aetna will cover 80 percent. That's 240 bucks we're responsible for, and were able to budget for it. How many times can I do such a thing? Why can't women's sexual healthcare be easy to find, and affordable?

On the elevator up, I'm curious about what I'll receive for this investment. The office I encounter resembles an art gallery with its cherry-red walls and contemporary oil paintings (pastoral scenes and conceptual cubes). I determine it's stylish here but not luxurious. What *is* luxe is the questionnaire I'm handed—twelve pages of medical history, most of it concerning sex. *Do you have pain or discomfort with penetration/intercourse? If so, when did you first start having discomfort with penetration/intercourse? Describe the pain on a scale of one to ten. Where, in the vagina or vulva, do you experience pain or discomfort? Have you ever had an orgasm? How often do you orgasm?*

Filling this out—seated in a blue leather chair, sipping mint tea they brought me—takes over an hour. They prepared me in advance. My hand gets tired but my brain is buzzing. I realize I never wrote it out this way, the entire chronology of my journey. I'm not alone in this detective work either. To my left is the doctor's inner chamber. I catch a glimpse of her scribbling on a massive oak desk. She looks a little like Meryl Streep, whom I've always imagined as a compassionate person.

Being here is already worth the money, I think as I complete the forms. Then they hand me a cover-up. A garment I've never gazed upon in this setting. It's a terry cloth robe, like at a spa.

Terry makes all the difference.

Once I'm in the examination room, this is especially true. Sitting on that horrifying table, waiting for the doc to knock-knock before she cranks me open, I'm not chilly like I usually am in this situation. In fact, I've left my pashmina on the chair. Toasty and serene, I select a *People* magazine from a rack on the peach-colored wall. I marvel at Queen Elizabeth's adorable little corgis like I'm waiting for a facial. It makes me scratch my head: *Why aren't all gynecologists using bathrobes in lieu of disposable paper? Is laundering more expensive than buying thousands of throw-away garments? They'd probably only need twenty bathrobes, total.* . . . Before I can crunch the numbers, Dr. Williams enters with my bulging medical history. She's wearing a sparkly blue necklace, which I try to focus on as she prepares the metal monster.

This apparatus is weirdly, shockingly, un-horrible—despite the vaginal pain I've been having. I think that's the robe helping too. Instead of a medieval torturer, Williams seems like a girlfriend who is only inadvertently pinching me. She is the fun Meryl with long hair in *Mamma Mia.*

"Okay, let's see what's going on here," announces the movie star between my knees.

The usual procedure continues, including clarification of what I put in the medical history. Eventually, she extracts the beast and does a manual exam.

"Do you feel that?" she asks, studying my eyes.

"Uh-huh," I reply, followed by, "Ow. Eesh."

"Exactly," she exclaims.

"Exactly?"

"Yeah. I thought so by your symptoms. Why don't you sit up?"

I do as she asks.

"You've got atrophy," she announces.

"Atrophy," I repeat.

"Do you know what atrophy is?"

"I think so." I pull my comfy robe belt tighter, trying to call up what I know about this word. Sixty-five-year-old Gina comes to mind, her warning at the Sex Brunch about menopausal dryness and pain. The Tantrika is in my psyche too, "It sounds like a shrinking vagina."

This must be a shrinking vagina.

Jeez, Francesca could have diagnosed this years ago. In a stream-of-conscious ramble, with nails dug into the exam table, I convey all these musings to my new gynecologist.

Dr. Williams, with a hand resting over her mouth, is glad I'm somewhat informed but she's surprised I don't know more—because I'm fifty-three. I'm surprised too. But I'm not even sure if my period has stopped or not. It's been four months since my last menses. "How do I know whether or not it's coming back?" I ask.

"Why don't you dress, and we can talk in my office?" she replies.

Once I'm seated in her large, artsy space—bookcases on three of the four cherry walls, more paintings, and even a Persian rug—she plops down in a chair behind her oak desk.

"So here's what I think is going on," she says like a confident scientist, but also a creative soul who likes deciphering the big picture. I half expect her to sing an ABBA song, swinging her blond hair. But it's the opposite. The content she releases has an unbearable melody.

This is what she tells me: my vaginismus has returned—even though it was, indeed, remedied by Stephanie, the PT. Vestibulitis is back too. Also, the lining of my vagina is inflamed and thin, a condition known as atrophy. But atrophy is part of larger changes called genitourinary syndrome of menopause (or GSM) that can cause infections, and bleeding, and narrowing, and more. Much more. I try taking it all in, but my skull feels like it ate too much. So I interrupt, emphasizing everything I've been doing to fix my genitals. The doctor says it doesn't matter. Middle age has gifted me new problems *and* the old ones exacerbated.

Suddenly, I smell coffee. The receptionist might be making some. I desperately want a big mug right now to caffeinate my comprehension because it seems like what this gynecologist is saying is that I'll never have great sex. Though I think she might be saying the opposite. I can't decide which! Either way, she has a remedy—estrogen. She recommends bioidentical hormones, which she prefers over a different kind of hormone. I can't decipher the two options because all I hear is "hormones."

"I can't take hormones," I retort. I complain that when I was twenty-four I went on birth control pills, which gave me high blood pressure. I swore after that I'd never mess with my endocrine system. "I don't want to use hormones," I reiterate.

"No one wants to use hormones," she replies. "The thing is, they work." She starts scribbling something on a pad—a prescription she will give to me, no doubt. She lets it sit in front of her as I come up with additional objections: some articles that came out a few years ago, linking estrogen and disease. "Doesn't estrogen increase your risk for breast cancer?" I ask accusingly, still not picking up the paper.

"A little," she says running her hands through her hair because she's frustrated with me. "But I think you'll really love it." Her shiny blue necklace is smiling at me.

"How long would I need to be on them?" I ask, yielding. Perhaps.

"Forever!" she answers. "This only gets worse with time." Then she comes around to my side of the desk. She sits on it and folds her arms. "Look," she says. "How old is your husband?"

"Sixty-two," I tell her.

"Okay. He's sixty-two." Her eyes drill into mine. "Is he still getting erections?"

"Yeah," I nod.

"All right.... Because ... a lot of women, when this develops, they just stop."

"My husband still gets erections," I assert, going along with her line of thinking—that phallus blood vessels are the rationale for a couple's physical intimacy. I do not question this. But then I do. It's like my head clears, even without that coffee.

Suddenly, I have woken up—once again—from the same phallus fallacy. Haven't the last five years been about rousing from this disempowering nightmare? "I want to have sex for me," I practically shout, "independent of my husband's erections."

"That's fine," she says before traveling back to the chair on her side of the desk. She's holding the prescription in her hand. "Whether you want to have sex for you, your husband, or both, your tissues need estrogen. That's just the way it is."

I take the prescription and leave.

Released to the Soho streets, I'm dizzy with confusion. *Should I take hormones? Or forbid them because they're dangerous? What about my life's dream of pleasure?* I cross intersections playing this out mentally, my head as congested as this New York City traffic. It's a miracle I don't get hit. I know where I'm going, though. Not the pharmacy. I'm on my way to La Perla, the Italian lingerie store.

This destination shop, upon arrival, is creamy-dreamy, just like Intimissimi. The signature scent is floral and flirty. I imagine corporate in Rome giving it a name like *Ti Voglio* ("I Want You"). Lace and silk underthings, lining both sides of the store, find their way to my fingertips. I love sniffing these items too. I pick up a simple bra and panty set in periwinkle. It costs more than my doctor's visit.

I am not in this league, I think.

At that moment, an energetic salesperson comes over. Her auburn hair gleams like the silver tile floors. Her white teeth are the brightest thing in here, contrasted with her burgundy lips.

"So beautiful, isn't it?" She's commenting on the periwinkle ensemble I'm still petting like it's my therapy dog. It must appear to the radiant employee that I'm contemplating extravagance. She starts telling me about the mailing list. If I give her my name, I'll be eligible for VIP previews with prosecco. There will be discounts and cupcakes, maybe a bit of cheese because that's what women like, a bit of cheese. Well, gals who do not yet count calories. Women not damaged from stress eating, the sun, *or* depleted ovaries.

I leave the store in a hurry because I don't belong in this club. I don't know if I ever will again.

On the bus home to DC, I record in my *Pleasure Plan* journal everything that went down, but I'm no longer in a daze. I keep writing until I reach a question: *What the hell do other women do with their menopause?*

Tips for *Your* Pleasure Plan

Something to Try:

If you suspect perimenopause or menopause might be implicated in your challenges, tell your doctor. If your physician doesn't seem comfortable talking about sexual dysfunction, go to another doc, and perhaps another, until you get someone who can really help. If you can, visit a physician who specializes in menopause, even for one appointment, as new remedies are being developed all the time.

Another avenue to explore if you're not happy with your medical care, or want another angle, is to get a prescription to see a pelvic floor physical therapist. These practitioners, who see people of all genders, can help with all kinds of pelvic pain.

Journal Prompts:

1. If you have female parts, are you getting as lubricated as before? Are you using antihistamines? Birth control pills? (These can cause dryness for premenopausal women.)

   _____

   _____

   _____

Journal Prompts (continued):

2. Did your problems begin after the age of forty?

   _____

   _____

   _____

3. Have you noticed any burning in or outside the vagina, especially during penetration?

   _____

   _____

   _____

4. Are you comfortable talking to your partner about these changes? If not, would you be willing to speak to a sex therapist, alone or with a partner? (See the Recommended Resources section in the Appendix for tips on how to find one.)

   _____

   _____

   _____

18

The Lemon

Back home after my doctor's appointment, and a long bus ride trying to analyze menopause data on the mini screen of my iPhone, I climb into bed—with statistics. Kurt's out of town on a business trip, so I ignore the late hour; I'm still wearing my jeans and navy blue cardigan. If someone were viewing me, they might think I'm comfortable—legs outstretched, laptop poised on thighs, four pillows behind my back—but they would be missing my knees, jammed together as I squint at what's in front of me.

According to a study affiliated with the Kinsey Institute, every year 7 percent of women past fifty give up on lovemaking. This figure keeps rising until, at age seventy, 54 percent of women have stopped engaging in intercourse, and 79 percent do not receive oral sex.

These data reflect what Gayle once told me about a study she conducted for her women's health organization, involving ladies in their seventies. When the discussion turned to physical intimacy, the septuagenarians went giddy. "You want to know the best part about being our age?" they gushed to my friend. "The best part is that your husband loses his erection. Finally, you can stop having sex."

From my vantage point, it's clear why these ladies revel in no nooky. It hurts! A favorite Buddhist teacher of mine, Pema Chodron, says that misery cracks a person's heart open. There's a benefit, though: a greater capacity for empathy and compassion. I don't know the effect of *vaginal* suffering, but right now I feel the ache of a billion pudenda filling up my pelvic bowl. Camaraderie doesn't help my situation though. Mine is still a dry and rigid vessel.

Does it have to be that way?

Behold Betty Dodson—at eighty-six, for fuck's sake. And what about Francesca? A different kind of woman in her seventies. The Kinsey report said 46 percent of gals in their seventh decade *are* doing it. Gayle should have polled those women.

Even so, I'm guessing what she would have found—these babes had zero disorders before the onset of atrophy. All the post-menopause sites I've investigated these past few hours have said the same thing: women *lose* elasticity, lubrication, and libido. What if she never had these to begin with? Or, she did have them, but only for a short time? What if, despite small gains, she possesses a precarious crotch?

These questions make me feel like I'm underwater, without an oxygen tank. I put my laptop down and turn on my side, curled into a tight little me. I feel restricted in my jeans and such, but I'm too exhausted to move. I'm wiped out by atrophy, and grilling, and studies, and buses, and doctors, and fear of breast cancer. It's time to numb myself through sleep.

I'm practically falling over by the time I open my overstuffed dresser, to pull out a pajama top. This simple action turns to confrontation. Suddenly, I'm staring at a chaotic collection of lingerie. I can't believe how many underthings I possess. It's as if someone entered my home while I was in New York, filling my private domain with abundance.

I should feel appreciative, but in my present state of mind, this steamy mélange seems silly and forced. I pick up a thong. Actually, I need to pull it apart from a tangle of butt floss. I start counting: hot pink, off-white, black, more black, lace, silk, poly, cotton, poly-cotton. Sixteen. Sixteen thongs!

I hate thongs.

When did I buy these? And why?

I trace the rationale. I started acquiring them when I became a yoga instructor thirteen years ago. I didn't want visible panty lines (or VPL). Somewhere, I got the memo: Beware of VPL. Heaven forbid the contours of my underwear be known. I went with this social pressure for years, until these garments started chafing.

I kept them, though, every piece—for turn-on. I discovered a formula. Ten minutes of titillation (and no more) prevented irritation. Those 600 seconds were fun, especially this past year when lovemaking improved.

Holding these thongs now in my hands, under a harsh overhead light, I imagine them on my degenerating genitals. Yuck. And do I honestly want apparel I only dress in for seconds at a time? I'm thinking of the seventies femmes in Gayle's report. They must have plenty of VPL. I bet they say things like, "Be sensible." That's going to be my mantra too: *Be sensible.* I throw all my thongs on the bed.

Next up is other ten-minute clothing. Crotchless lace undies in gaudy scarlet. Bras that match them, with a slit down the middle so nipples poke out. I've got two of these sets! I think back to the last time I wore either. It was right before I saw Francesca. I was still trying to get excited. And I did feel slutty in these ensembles, deliciously. But now sensuality is on a rug that's been pulled from under me. *I started too late*, I say to myself. I say it again as my eyes water and my nose drips. I grab a tissue but do not stop the purge.

A mauve miniskirt with hooks for attaching stockings? It has to go. What about a lime bustier? I toss both these garments on the growing pile taking over my comforter. When I get to the Intimissimi pieces I purchased on my honeymoon—three elaborate lingerie families, made up of panties, camisoles, push-up contraptions, and slips—I discard these too because I see now what I knew back then: these garments are, comprehensively, scratchy. Scratchy does not match a precarious crotch.

I started too late; I keep saying to myself. Then I pick up an item I bought in my twenties—a black velvet bra. This was one of the things I wore when I'd walk down the streets of New York, wanting to be sexy. It didn't work. Not enough. But it did make me feel beautiful. I get lost for a moment stroking the luxurious fabric. I hold this brassiere up to my still-runny nostrils. It smells like lemon verbena because I keep soaps in that drawer. I love this bra, but it's impractical like the rest. I haven't worn it in years. I place it on the pile, topping it off.

Moving the expulsion along, I grab a plastic trash bag from the kitchen, a million-gallon one. I dump my intimates inside, thinking about tomorrow when I'll donate this bag, or take it to the trash bin in my apartment's basement.

When I behold my revised dresser, I can't believe its spaciousness. It's like a dream. The one where you discover home expansion you never knew existed. Gigantic rooms that smell of wind and cinnamon. Kurt and I talked about moving to a bigger apartment one day. We even vied for one in our building, but our modest offer got outbid. All of a sudden, discarding seems symbolic. It is gliding me into a different life. Who could I have been if I hadn't spent the last five years chasing a lovemaking fantasy?

Who can I be now?

Once I change and get under the covers, I spread out in the burgundy sheets. And you know what? My bed seems bigger too. But that's only because no one else is here. I start wondering, with a dry throat, what will happen once my husband returns. A memory trickles in, an encounter with my friend Sally.

I was visiting her and her spouse, Bill, ten years before, at their beach house in Delaware. We were all putting away groceries we'd purchased for the weekend. I paused to watch my gorgeous friend, a six-foot-tall tennis player. At fifty-three, Sally had retained her youthful athleticism. When she reached into the cabinets, her tight, sports top crept up, revealing six-pack abs. "You're so sexy," I gushed.

"You're right. I *am* sexy," she boasted with hands on hips. She posed like I was taking photos. "Sexy, but nothing else," she added before going back to unpacking. "I'm done."

"Done with what?" I asked.

"With fooling around!" she responded, emphatically.

I still wasn't comprehending. "With sex?"

"Yes, with sex." She furrowed her brow like she was worried about my mental function. Sally explained: she now lived a platonic life with her husband, who was also storing away food in the kitchen. He was standing right next to us.

"What does Bill think?" I asked, giving him a wink because surely his wife was kidding.

"I told Bill. I'm done." She was staring at only me and my low IQ, not her husband. "We don't need it," she declared. Then she locked eyes with Bill. "We have laughs," she said, bursting into peels of it.

I looked at Bill, who was chuckling along. Then he shut a cabinet with a little too much force. He quickly left the room.

A decade later, in my near-empty bed, I can still feel the slam of those cupboards, the closing of that door.

What *will* take place when my husband returns?

I'm suddenly sweaty, so I kick off the covers. Sally's solution brings on a hot flash, or at least I suspect that's what this is. I feel dipped in clammy, sticky moisture. As I pull off my PJ bottoms, I mentally play out a scenario: Kurt being in Bill's shoes . . . slamming cabinets.

I know those slams. They represent a chasm I've been running from for five years. Kurt being angry and hurt, crying, "Why do you keep rejecting me?"

This is the loneliness haunting me my whole life—until I met my husband and found a way to be intimate. This is the rift that makes my bones fragile with aching alienation.

I can't do what Sally did. I can't! But this leaves me only one option. "Just. Have. Sex."

That's what the hypnotist told me at the beginning of my odyssey. "Just have sex" is how you stop your husband from leaving you. Of course it is. Except for a few recent years, it's how I always kept a man (or tried to) because this is what women's bodies are designed for. My mother taught me all about it—what you do to survive.

Isn't that what happened with the Cadillac?

My mother took me to the dealership to get it. I think I was eight years old. The whole way over she chattered nonstop, excited. Like all our cars, this would be a pre-owned auto, which she pronounced OW-*to*. But finally, we would own a vehicle that worked.

When we got there, she showed me the set of wheels. It was stupendously white with red trim. A 1970 Coupe Deville, that car was enormous. I kept circling the cool rear fins, the fancy front grill. Then Mom brought me back to the vehicle we arrived in, warning me to stay inside. She needed to negotiate a price.

Trapped in our beige, beat-up Pontiac, I found the temperature stifling. It vaporized fruits and vegetables rotting in the trunk, a norm for my mom. I kept the windows closed, regardless. I didn't want to hear anything. I kept biting the inside of my lip, which tasted like my pizza lunch. In my school bag was a Barbie doll with matted hair. I'd brought a comb and crochet needles, a ball of yarn. I could make a doll hat if I wanted. Instead, I kept moving from the front seat to the back, and vice versa. *Something was going on in there.*

I don't know how I knew, but I did. I saw flashes of a conference table, surrounded by men in boxy blue suits. I must have seen an image like this on TV. I placed my mom in this room but went no further. *Still, I knew what she was doing.*

I started feeling sick from the pizza cheese, and knots of worry in my stomach. I lay down in the back seat, but now the images came faster. An onslaught of things I tenaciously didn't comprehend: so many blue jackets, and pants, and white shirts. They leered at my mother, who had exposed herself. Jabbing one another in the side, the men snickered, "Hey, look at that."

It felt like years before my mother came out. She got in the driver's seat and started the engine. I stayed in the back seat but could see her creased forehead in the rearview mirror as she reversed the car, in a hurry. When we were out of the parking lot, she said, "Okay. Now we have a car that's not a lemon." Her face appeared as if she had sucked on the lemon that was our *old* car.

After that day, I paid closer attention to my mother's sources of income. Much of it was through hairdressing. She'd go to ladies' homes, which seemed safe to me. Other times, she disappeared into the houses of elderly men. She said that she cleaned their apartments, shopped for them, and took these guys to the doctor. I suspected *other* pursuits but didn't have the nerve to bring it up. Even half thinking about what might be going on made me ill and antsy like that day at the dealership.

There was a slew of these guys, one after the other. For a few years, she cared for two simultaneously. My father knew about this employment, the general scope of it; I'm not sure if he peeked under this rock. She met her "old guys" at a Senior Center she frequented. I think she went there specifically to find them—single elders who had a bursting bank account and no one to nurture them.

Whatever the arrangement, the men were complicit—and smitten. "Your mother is quite a woman." That's what Jerry would say, endlessly, in his Bronx accent. His bald pate and tattooed arms made him look exactly like Popeye. He'd tap my shoulder like I was a deaf little ingrate: "Did you hear what I said? Your mother is quite a woman."

I always changed the subject. It might take days for me to shake off the shame that had caved in my chest.

One day, when I was twenty-four, my mother unveiled her secrets. We were driving to her house and had just stopped at a traffic light. A moment before I had been complaining about my day job doing medical transcription. Suddenly, my mother blurted out, "Money, money, money. There's *a lot* I've done for money.... Do you think I liked touching Morty's balls?"

I instantly pictured Morty. He was slight with countable strands of silver hair. His entire head and body (what I could see of it) were covered in crusty liver spots. I tried not to think about where else that crustiness lived.

In spite of cringing, I was relieved these facts were out in the open. A moment later, I wanted nothing to do with this discussion. However, Mom was staying on topic: "Do you think I liked it?"

"Of course not," I said a tad sarcastically because I thought she might be chastising me. After all, I had been whining about a job that wasn't awful, not comparatively. But when I glanced at my mother's jewel-quality orbs, I grasped they were speaking to me on their own, communicating in code. I couldn't decipher the message, though. What I received was glowing intensity that burnt my retina. This sometimes was the case with her and her eyes—too much fucking light. I turned my head to scan the passing Burger King, the supermarket, the mechanic shops beyond it.

"Do you understand?" she asked as she drove.

"Yeah, I do," I said without looking at her.

When we got to her house and she had parked, she bore into me again. "Do you?"

I noticed, only then, I was trembling, and had been since she first told me. I sighed and gave her my full attention, surrendering to the green mystery of her soul. I saw exploding bombs, and shiny gold caps, extracted from corpses. I saw sunlight reflected off Nazi boots. I saw belt buckles.

"You did what you needed to," I said to stop the onslaught of light now burning my skin. Also, I *did* understand. That's what men were like. Pigs groping the women who cleaned their houses. They preyed on females who thought abuse was normal. Of course, my mother sold her body. She didn't think she deserved better.

❋

Twenty-nine years later, recalling my mother's relationship with sex, in my own red bed, my heart bleeds for the unique suffering of her life. Cleaning the toilets of horrid old men, and fucking them on the side. . . . It crushes me with sadness, especially since I never talked to my mother this way again. A few years later, after having lunch with me, she sped off in a car bought for her by another of these "patrons." For months, she had been bone weary, working for Jerry while driving back and forth to see my dad who had been put in a nursing home. Mom had a fatal heart attack on the highway. Lack of pleasure was, undeniably, a factor in her death.

However, pleasure was also a factor in her life!

I sit up and hug my knees to my chest. The chandelier on the ceiling grabs my attention. Though its light is harsh, it sparkles just the same. Didn't my mother's transactions with decrepit, randy guys have power in it? It had *chutzpah*. Chutzpah is Yiddish for courage or determination. Everything was taken from her but she was determined to get it back, for me.

Through me.

Ballet recitals and velvet jewelry boxes. Singing lessons and silk chiffon shorts. Tap dancing, jazz, and acting. She charged these on credit cards she begged my father to pay off. She purchased these with heads she saturated in peroxide. She bought my future with Morty's balls.

Giving up on myself—on my life force—is not an option.

I am the juice of those damaged lemons.

I am my mother's lemonade.

Tips for *Your* Pleasure Plan

Something to Try:

Make a list of partners that you feel contributed to your sexual healing. When you're done, take stock of your journey and the people that helped. If no one has taken on this role for you, are there friends who have helped you on the sexual healing journey you've been on all along?

Journal Prompts:

1. What messages about sex did you get from your family?

   _____

   _____

   _____

2. Which family messages are useful in your life? Which family messages are not useful?

   _____

   _____

   _____

3. Does having a healthy sex life enhance your life? If so, how?

   _____

   _____

   _____

19

What Is Pleasure?

The next morning, I wake up in love. I'm in love with a person who's been fighting for colors, erotic zeniths, and closeness. I am in love with a warrior.

Before I fell asleep last night, I committed myself to a lifelong fight, taking stock of my army—all the healers I've seen these five years of searching. They're not a unified force yet; that's for sure. But they could be, provided I train these women for a mission, a single mission of keeping me connected to Eros, for life.

Thank God it's Saturday, and Kurt is still away. There's time to accomplish a feat this weekend I have not yet attempted. I've got to synthesize what I've learned. This involves combing through every inch of *The Pleasure Plan*—a formidable task. You see, over time, my one blank book expanded into three identical diaries filled with notes, observations, snippets of conversation, statistics, reflections, and remedies. On each respective cover, I've written *Book One, Book Two,* and *Book Three*. This is my oeuvre, my bible.

An hour later, after pushing my coffee table forward, I sit on the rug with my back against the sofa, journals scattered around my toes.

Kombucha is also standing by. Then, with fingertips and tears, with fermented tea and two kinds of readers, I begin studying my odyssey.

Right away, I find it's in my ears as well as my ink. That's how I best remember these goddesses.

"Chicks need their own erections," says Betty Dodson in her gruff, maternal voice.

"Yes, engorgement is important," chimes in Francesca. "But don't forget safety. Don't forget Surrender Breath."

"Kegels," calls out Stephanie, who also yells, "dilators!"

Released from the binding of the diaries—as well as time and space—these females surround me, for hours. It's a chorus of healing mamas, snapping and swaying around my apartment. "You found agency," belts the trauma therapist. A bit later, a duo, comprised of EFT and EMDR, sings me a lullaby with a single verse: *Regulate your nervous system.* The hypnotist interrupts this song, to chant her filthy phrases.

I listen to this chorus throughout the morning and afternoon, scribbling notes. It's hard not to notice that, lovely as they are, these voices do not blend. I keep waiting for a summative presence to show up. The Ghost of Vagina Christmas Past!

No one of this scope arrives, so I keep writing. By seven in the evening, mostly glued to the same patch of floor, my hand almost falling off, I'm about to quit. But then I hear a small voice—it might be my own—that says: *Go get the garbage.*

Not the kitchen trash, but the Hefty bag still sitting in a corner of my bedroom. Inside, tangled in a heap, is the black velvet bra I discarded the night before. Of all the rejected lingerie, I don't know why I'm summoned to this piece. I take it out, nonetheless. After removing my yoga pants and sweatshirt, I put it on.

It just so happens our boudoir has a giant Victorian mirror my mother passed down to me. Four feet high and two feet across, with a mahogany frame composed of intricate carvings (roses, gardenias, and other flora), it resembles an object from a Disney movie: *mirror, mirror on the wall.* I stand before this magic reflection in my aging bra, which shockingly fits. The shape, still perfect for my breasts, is actually a balconette. This realization makes my mouth upturn like each half-circle of the underwire.

There are so many lovers for whom I've donned this intimate. But now I wear it for myself. Feeling confident—I mean, this ancient garment is still wearable, after many pounds and decades—I look in my fairy-tale glass and ask: *Do I behold the fairest of them all?*

"No!" answers my reflection with a smirk, followed by: *Are you kidding me?*

Even so, I know that I behold the fullest.

I think of the eighty-eight keys Mama Gena talked about. I can see many of them in my mirror. This body of mine represents many brilliant notes, reclaimed. Yet, other keys are chipped, yellowed, or broken. Yeah, they're broken. But taking in my visage—my plush pretty bra, my (un-matching) polka dot panties, and all my hideous dysfunctions—I am stunning. Maybe the gaze that has always mattered most is my own.

I dance a little for myself, even though I'm not young, liquid movements taking over my limbs. In the midst, insight washes over me: understanding.

After three decades, I finally comprehend the difference between wanting to be sexy and wanting sex. It's simple. So simple that I feel dumb not having put this together before. A quest for sexiness is, indeed, a journey for wholeness, as I deciphered at the Mama Gena event. With radical acceptance—like right at this moment—I am equipped for authentic decision-making: to engage physically, to not engage physically, or to get a gelato. Desire is a longing for pleasure, inspired by truth.

Standing in my balconette, shimmying for myself, I ask the woman before me: *What do you desire, my love?*

The answer comes right away.

A trousseau would be nice. . . .

Currently, my "trousseau" is an underwear blob stuffed in a garbage bag. I empty these items back on the bed. What a pile of confusion. No, I won't keep everything. But I'd like the opportunity to prune, thoughtfully. And what I keep will be meaningfully arranged.

The next day, I go hunting. Sunday is a horrible day to hit up IKEA as well as the Container Store, but I do it anyway—without success. Driving home, on a lark, I stop at a used furniture store I like to rummage through sometimes, its basement crammed with junk but also, occasionally, treasures. My instinct is correct. Downstairs, amidst bowls, bicycle pumps, and army jackets that make me sneeze, I find perfection—a box that once held a tea set, in black lacquer. It's so freakin' shiny.

When I get it home, I clean it thoroughly and place key items inside, leaving room for estrogen cream, which I've started reading up on. From what I can tell, hormones appear safe for many people. Yes, replacement therapy will go into my hope chest.

My hope chest.

I like this term for trousseau. It makes me think I'm doing all of this for my chest, my own heart. A way of keeping myself in love.

A few weeks later, while Kurt is at work, I open my fab lacquer box, taking out the accumulated contents. New to this collection is a bag of chocolates with a ribbon. I told the salesperson it was a present because it is.

Then I get into bed. Propped up on a plethora of pillows behind me, listening to the summer birds romantically call to each other, I pray for synthesis. I think I now know what that means. It's not, ultimately, a consensus among my practitioners. It's a meeting with my demons, sexually. It's an orgy with monsters.

One at a time, I invite my sexual problems into the bed.

Low Libido is first. I ask her what she'd like. Right away, pedantically, she directs me to the new *DSM*, emphasizing that arousal grows out of desire. She needs me to grasp this, as well as the toll of my anxiety—how my lack of carnal appetite is often due to stress. "Take more baths," she tells me. And try Sensate Focus." She's talking about a Masters and Johnson technique whereby touch is done for its own sake. "Do these and then see how you feel," she instructs before sauntering away. And despite her name, there's plenty of libido in her hips.

At that moment, Arousal bursts in. Though some days he likes to take his time, calibrating the balance between accelerator and brake, today he is demanding. "My hard-on is important," he tells me. He starts talking about stuff: fantasy, music, toys, black velvet bras, erotica, chocolates, and variety—tons of variety. When I ask him, "What else?" He says, "Surprise me." Rather than leave, he sits in a corner so he can watch the other action. He's always interested in new action.

My ugly creatures of pelvic pain arrive just then, craving their own caresses and remedies. Vaginismus longs for dildos, estrogen, lube, and moisture cream twice a week. Vestibulitis digs estrogen too, and perhaps a dab of testosterone. Deep Thrusting Pain just wants communication with my husband, making sure positions and rhythms work for all concerned. Once they're sated, these pain demons exit, leaving room in the bed for my sixth paramour—Orgasm.

Orgasm is not interested in categories and labels. It is more fluid. "Stop trying to classify my pleasure," it asserts, emphasizing it's interested in only two questions: "What do I want?" and "Was I satisfied?"

I do *not* invite my abusers to my lovefest. However, I do think of the main spot where I was molested—the garage. Over the last few months, I discovered a whole new relationship to this memory. I don't know if it was taking the trip to Brooklyn, writing about it, or talking up my play, but every time I think of that horror house, my mind only conjures the remodeled office, IKEA furniture abounding.

But I'm not fooled.

The old location is waiting for me, like all my interior beasts and devils, like all my naughty-in-a-bad-way tendencies—fried food, over-spending and numbing out. I want to be free of destructive forces, permanently. But how can I? At this moment, my tight neck, resting upon four pillows, shouts that I've not been consistent with the PT exercises I'm supposed to be doing for my *upper* body. When I do these exercises, my neck is great; when I don't, it's achy. Good wiring is possible, but it must be maintained. Constantly.

Considering this example, I glance out the window in my bedroom and see the same sooty grey brick wall as always. It occurs to me— perhaps for the very first time—that being erotically unencumbered is *not* a state I will ever reach. After five years of climbing, I will never scale that height.

I run my hands over the shiny lacquer box sitting next to me on the bed before eating the last of the four chocolates in the bag. I'm letting it sink in: I will never be fully healed. But I *am* working on

Eros—which might be enough. I think it is. *Working on Eros is what makes me a sexual person.*

I've been a sexual person all along.

As my private time comes to a close (Kurt will be home soon), I realize I need sessions like this one if I want to stay healthy. Solo time I'll have to negotiate with my partner. How will I manage this? Will I tell him? I decide I will because I want sixty minutes, weekly. Sixty minutes to keep my PC muscles—and arousal—toned. Three hundred and sixty seconds to engage with a demon or two while conducting radiance research: recovery and discovery. In a nod to *The Pleasure Plan*, I christen this practice The Pleasure Hour.

Can I keep these appointments with myself?

I have to.

It might be the most important thing I'll ever do.

Tips for *Your* Pleasure Plan

Something to Try:

Ideas for a Pleasure Minute: Using one of your five senses, notice something delightful or interesting. It could be the taste of coffee still sitting on your taste buds, the scent of that lovely shampoo you used that day. Now, move to another sense, searching and then finding something pleasing. Keep going until you're buzzing with full sensory fun.

For Pleasure Hour ideas, see the Recommended Resources section in the Appendix.

Journal Prompts:

1. What could you do for one minute a day that would connect you to your erotic self?

    _____

    _____

    _____

2. What could you do for one hour a week that would connect you to your erotic self?

    _____

    _____

    _____

3. Which minute of the day would you choose for your Pleasure Minute? Can you schedule this now?

    _____

    _____

    _____

4. Which hour of the week would you choose for your Pleasure Hour? Could you schedule this now?

    _____

    _____

    _____

20

The Trousseau

It's a Sunday evening in June. On this balmy night, Kurt and I lounge in coordinated terry-cloth robes in front of a faux fireplace—the centerpiece of our new two-bedroom condo. Miraculously, a nice couple accepted a real-estate offer we made. As soon as we moved into this apartment (almost twice the size of our previous abode), we went in search of an antique mantel. We painted it white and propped it against a long wall in our humongous (for us) living room. Inside the arch, on the gleaming hardwood floor, we placed a mirrored tray with six pillar candles.

Two years have passed since I purchased the trousseau and implemented the Pleasure Hour, which I've kept consistent. Much has come into existence during this time. Most relevantly, I became a sexuality educator. I needed a way to share what I'd discovered—and continue to discover—through my pleasure-healing odyssey. I combine this work with speaking, writing, and performing. In the wake of #MeToo—which has encouraged so many survivors to speak out and has inspired women to demand bliss as well as fair treatment—I've become very busy. Kurt's career has heated up too. After retiring from his job, he started a consulting firm that helps organizations prevent sexual harassment and other misconduct. Even professionally, my love and I are intertwined.

But now our candles need to be lit. We both rise to find fire. He likes matchbooks; I prefer long wooden sticks. An argument ensues about which is better. Wicks get ignited nonetheless. My husband and I settle back into our blaze-gazing nest, comprised of yoga mats, a red velvet blanket, and cushions from our sofa—in teal and magenta.

"So what are you in the mood for?" Kurt asks, leaning on an elbow, his legs extended, like a mischievous sultan.

I marvel at flecks of humor and curiosity dancing in his two irises. "I'm not sure yet," I say. Then I notice the incense. He must have begun burning it a moment ago. I close my eyes to float into the smoke.

There are so many ways this can go. All of them involve my trousseau. That shiny lacquer chamber continues to grow its contents. Most recently, I added a new lube that's fab. It complements the twin creams also in my sex box—estrogen and hyaluronic acid (HA). I've prepped for this rendezvous by employing both these assistants (estrogen yesterday and HA the day before). Scheduling lovemaking has helped me organize this regimen.

Yet lotions and potions, plus titillation tools, are only the physical manifestation of my hope chest, which also includes nonphysical things—everything I've absorbed since I began *The Pleasure Plan* in August 2011. Strategies and habits are equally, and carefully, folded inside.

Spontaneously, I pluck one from the collection. "Here's what I'm in the mood for," I say. Scooting forward, I nestle my body into my mate's contours, lifting my chin. What I'm after is a kiss. As our lips meet, waves of heat and hunger-passion awaken my yoni, my heart, and the part of me that talks to stars. In other words, it's just like in the movies. No, better, much better, because we worked to create this perfect smooch. I grin, thinking of the whole process.

✳

It started with our adventure seeing the Tantrika—as a couple. We both wanted better skills for communicating what we liked and didn't like. For me, after learning to voice my need for pleasure, expressing my *dis*pleasure seemed the final, final frontier.

At Francesca's, after removing every stitch, we hopped on the golden comforter, embracing with embarrassment. But gazing into my partner's face, I saw his pride: *Look how far we've traveled together.* This intimacy was interrupted by our hostess, who scooted next to us on the bed. "Show me," she whispered. "How do you kiss normally?"

On command, awkwardly, we made out, holding each other's backs before parting.

"How was it?" asked Francesca with Mediterranean candor.

"Grrreat," said Kurt, like he was Tony the Tiger.

"It *was* great," I repeated, pulling my eyes from his so I could shift them to Francesca, with whom I stayed. "But," I continued, "I want…It would be nice if he pressed more.…I mean sometimes, not always, I don't love the way he kisses me."

Tentatively, I turned to my husband, my epidermis flushed in fear. He was frowning, confused. "You don't like the way I kiss?"

I shook my head no, feeling my jagged breath.

Francesca swooped in for a rescue. "What is it you don't like, Laura?"

Quietly, I advocated for more lip and less tongue. Avoiding the word *sloppy* was difficult; I wasn't successful.

"My kisses are sloppy?" my guy exclaimed.

"A little," I told him with nervous energy now blushing my whole body. But power was underneath this pink. I began to grasp that, going forward, I could request an optimum, sensuous experience. I could ask him to brush his teeth, clip his nails, or not wear the undies with holes. If his privates were not washed to my satisfaction, I was allowed to demand (politely) a do-over. Could I really be that brazen?

"You must!" urged the Tantrika. She then advised: "First we praise what we *do* like. We validate our lover's needs." Kurt spontaneously modeled this: "I love kissing you. *You* know that. And I hear what you're saying about lips. But I need more tongue."

In other words, he didn't like my make-out style either.

Ouch.

But also, Ha. We laughed wildly—me, my sexual partner, and our coach.

Before we ended our session, Francesca emphasized how Kurt and I could be healers for each other. She showed him Surrender Breath, to chill out my nervous system. She taught *me* a technique to ground him in happiness, pressing on his perineum while saying loving phrases. These methods of connection, she stressed, were a microscopic taste of the vast union tantra has in mind.

Released into the sunshine, strolling toward the nearby Hudson River, Kurt and I pledged to uphold Francesca's vision for our lives—healing each other. I felt some of that potential at the river itself, where cerulean sky brightened black water. I pointed out a jutting strip of land in the distance. It was the peninsula where I grew up. We could see it and its implications: Gravesend Bay becoming the Hudson River, becoming the Atlantic Ocean, connecting to all the fluid on our planet. A phrase came to mind, the same one as when I was on the beach in Brooklyn that day. *None of us are just the size of ourselves.*

✳

Almost a year later, in our living room, embracing Kurt, I feel the amplitude of merging. Then he breaks the hug. "So I found something I want to show you," he says with a mischievous twinkle. "It's right here." From under a pile of cushions, he produces his iPad, which he burrows into.

I grin at Kurt and his plethora of devices.

"I downloaded a book," he tells me.

"A book?" A rosebud pops open in my heart.

"I have to find it," he says, scrolling.

Kurt has become accustomed to my need for novelty. I'm used to his requirements too. We're both adjusting to what's been added to our trousseau these past two months.

When I first seized upon the image of a hope chest, in the lead-up to my honeymoon, I wanted the dream offered a nineteenth-century woman traveling to her marriage bed. Arriving with her would be a cedar trunk she'd open when she longed for the fragrance of faith. Perfect years ahead would be stitched into starched nightgowns, crinolines, and tablecloths.

I've come to understand how incomplete this concept is. Everything goes into the sex box we bring to our partnership. Each person brings a separate container that's yoked to a mate's—forming a trunk of wanted and unwanted cargo. In this latter category is the reality I now share with my spouse. Despite the charm of our fireplace interlude, these last weeks have been hard.

On April 4, 2019, during the writing of this book, Kurt was diagnosed with pancreatic cancer, the fourth-largest killer worldwide. Only 9 percent of people with this diagnosis live beyond five years.

That's because it's mostly found at stage IV. Blessedly, Kurt's was discovered early. His trust in doctors is what saved him. After upper-abdominal distress refused to dissipate, he relentlessly sought medical help. Eventually, doctors found a tumor before it metastasized. Also, though not usually the case, my husband was fully operable. He emerged from surgery with a positive prognosis. Under his sexy-clean white robe is a five-inch scar running up his abdomen.

I loosen his belt just then to examine the four incisions we're still keeping an eye on, though they're mostly mended now. As I scrutinize these sites, Kurt continues looking through his iPad while also caressing my hair. In days, he'll start chemotherapy—some of the strongest and least targeted in the world. Poison will be added to our trousseau.

The thought of chemo eating up my husband's vibrant cells is filth soiling the pristine fabrics of my imagination. I don't want cancer, or its chemicals, to be part of my life—or my bedroom. I also would not have chosen three perverts using my small body for their own gratification, damaging me for decades. One's hope chest houses the gamut. But what comes out of that dark, mixing space is our own choice. My current choice is staying where I am in front of the fireplace, with candles aflame, incense still wafting. My choice is to adjust our romance to these circumstances, to continue making love.

"Here it is," Kurt announces. He's found the downloaded book. It turns out to be a self-help tome by Xaviera Hollander. She penned one of the lustful tomes I uncovered in my father's drawer when I was twelve. This memory cracks us both up.

"You're so sweet," I tell him, followed by many rounds of "Schmookie," "My Schmookie," and "You wanna be my Schmookie?"

"You know me; I find things," he says with a proud grin.

It's true. He's always digging up new adventures. I am too. For this reason, we've decided *The Pleasure Plan* will never really end.

After perusing the Hollander book, we decide to try it another time.

"Why don't we just get naked," Kurt suggests.

We remove our robes and stand looking at each other.

I trace the four scars with my fingers, just as he's been tracing *my* scars for the ten years of our marriage. Almost ten years.

Finally, we inch toward each other until we are flesh to flesh.

"What's next?" my beloved whispers in my ear.

So many possibilities.

"Let's figure it out," I conclude.

And that's what we do. We figure it out.

Together.

Appendix

How to Create Your Own Pleasure Plan

The Pleasure Plan Process

Healing your sexuality can be scary, but it just might blossom every aspect of your life. In the following pages, I offer resources featured in my book—and beyond. As you can see from my story, progress might not be very linear. Be gentle with yourself. If you've not seen a physician, start there. Involving a therapist in your process—especially a sex therapist or someone who is comfortable talking about these matters—is also a smart idea.

Here's a rough schema that can help you begin your own Pleasure Plan process, but feel free to improvise. Visit *LauraZam.com/My PleasurePlan* for a free Pleasure Plan kit that goes into detail about each of the steps below.

1. **Create** a pleasure goal.
2. **Dedicate** a blank journal or unused notebook for this journey.
3. **Organize** your book into five sections: (1) thoughts on why this goal is important; (2) a list of experts you could see, or others you could talk to; (3) your doubts and fears; (4) a challenge

(or antidote) for each doubt and fear; (5) notes on your visits with experts.

4. **Implement** a healing habit. A Pleasure Hour is an example of a healing habit. So is daily meditation, even for one minute.

5. **Share** a portion of your journal with someone. It doesn't have to be verbatim; it could just be an insight you recorded. A therapist is a good choice for someone with whom you'll share. Other choices include a group of people who have a similar problem (think: blog, an affinity group meeting, a post on social media). The public aspect of the Pleasure Plan process can help you root out shame. Sharing also stimulates innovative thinking and solutions.

My Curative Adventures

1. Medical Doctors (Gynecology)

I would start a sexual healing journey by seeing a doctor. If possible, try to find one that specializes in your problem. It's also great if this person has solid training in human sexuality. As you can see from my journey, only one of my gynecologists was helpful. See How to Find a Sexual Healing Expert in this Appendix.

2. Sex Therapy

Since the sex therapist I contacted wouldn't see me, my story does not include much about this modality. Don't be misled by this lack of attention. Sex therapy can be a fantastic way to treat sexual problems, including all the relationship aspects. Sex therapists are licensed therapists with specialized, very rigorous, sexuality education. Aside from a medical doctor, I would start here with treatment, especially if psychological factors are complicating the problem.

3. **Vaginal Weights**

There are many devices that will help you strengthen the pelvic floor. They are all best used with guidance from a doctor or pelvic floor physical therapist. In many instances, like my own, strengthening is not recommended until tightness is mitigated.

4. **Healing Art Project**

Making art about my problems is what allowed me to get unstuck. I encourage you to try something creative if, similarly, you feel paralyzed. If you don't think you have artistic talent, even better! Do it for yourself—for processing and expression. A drawing, a poem, a story, a song...

5. **Cognitive Behavioral Therapy (CBT)**

CBT is a type of psychotherapy that focuses on changing negative thinking or behavior patterns. Usually, this type of therapy is very goal oriented. For instance, CBT is commonly used to overcome phobias. In my opinion, CBT can be a wonderful treatment for sexual problems (it can help you rewire); however, this modality is best integrated into a larger framework that includes a medical diagnosis and therapeutic strategy administered by someone with vast knowledge of your issue, like a sex therapist.

6. **Hypnosis**

Hypnosis is a CBT technique. It can surely have a place in sexual healing, especially with regard to anxiety-reduction. I would not recommend hypnosis as a first stop regarding painful sex (that's what I did). These conditions often reflect an underlying medical condition that needs proper diagnosing. In other words, if you have pain, it's probably not in your head; it's in your vagina (or penis, etc.).

7. **Sex Brunch**

Gathering friends to talk about sex was frightening, but it helped me get comfortable asking questions and seeking help. If you'd like to try this yourself, you don't need a formal event. Just grab a friend or two, and maybe some bagels. (See How to Host Your Own Sex Brunch.)

8. **Role Play/Fantasy**

Once I got my physical problems under control, I set about developing my erotic mind. Role play and fantasy were key. Both of these can help you restart a stalled mojo—by increasing arousal, ramping up novelty, and injecting fun. I'm a big fan of these techniques.

9. **Couples Retreat**

If you're in a relationship, I highly recommend some form of intimacy workshop, course, or retreat that you can do with your partner. This experience can give you and your person a shared set of skills. The retreat Kurt and I attended is *IntimacyRetreats.com*.

10. **Tantra**

Tantra is a big topic, and there are many access points. I recommend your own exploration. Under Recommended Resources, I've included a good place to start.

11. **Emotional Freedom Technique (EFT)**

This technique helps a person calm the nervous system vis-à-vis disturbing memories or thoughts. You can find many terrific free videos on YouTube that show you how to use it.

12. **Exposure Therapy/Prolonged Exposure (PE)**

Exposure therapy is the larger category that PE falls under. Essentially, all of these techniques desensitize us to disturbing stimuli. By exposing us gradually, or repeatedly (or both), we are no longer activated. Exposure therapy can also be used with physical responses. Dilator use, for instance, is a type of exposure therapy—dilators desensitize the freak-out response of our pelvic floor. Talk to a therapist about possibilities in this realm.

13. **Story Therapy**

Story therapy is a form of intervention that helps a person reframe the stories they tell themselves about their lives, or about certain experiences. This modality has a relationship with narrative therapy, developed by Michael White and David Epston. Though it wasn't my original goal, the visit I took to the house where I was abused turned into a story therapy experience—sort of. Since this was done without a therapist, it was more of an intuitive, self-help endeavor. But it worked! For tips on how to rewrite your own story, visit my website.

14. **Trauma Therapy**

Many therapists specialize in trauma, which is terrific. If you have sexual trauma, and you have not already worked successfully with a trauma specialist, I would recommend finding one you click with. Make sure this person knows about sex and sexual recovery. I would also recommend getting a medical diagnosis in conjunction with any psychotherapy you're undergoing. Sometimes therapists will try to treat sexual problems from a psychological perspective (their specialty) without a medical intervention. A multidisciplinary approach is best.

15. Public Speaking

I can't speak highly enough about talking openly about your awful sex life. For centuries, women forced themselves to endure excruciating or lousy sex. Survivors of sexual trauma often feel shame about the ways harm has affected our bodies. Those seeking sexual healing can help society—including healing professionals—respond to our needs by speaking up. We might also help a friend who is going through something similar.

16. Physical Therapy

Pelvic floor physical therapists are the unsung heroes and sheroes of the sexual healing world. This kind of PT can address a host of issues, including incontinence, erectile dysfunction, painful vaginal sex, post-pregnancy pelvic weakness, increased need to urinate, and bowel dysfunction. If you're not sure if your doctor knows enough about your condition, try getting a prescription to see one of these experts.

17. Dilators

Dilators can help with painful sex, narrowing of the vagina, vestibular burning, male-to-female gender reassignment surgery, and other situations and conditions. Since I began my journey, more companies have entered this market, offering a greater variety of these products. For instance, you can now find soft silicone dilators, and even dilators that vibrate. See my website for options.

18. **Mama Gena's School of Womanly Arts**

Since I dedicate a whole chapter to this experience I'll just add here that Mama Gena has written a few excellent books, and she offers a variety of courses. She's worth investigating, in my opinion.

19. **Orgasmic Meditation**

This experience gets only a short mention in my story due to space. Essentially, it's a way of combining mindfulness and sensual stroking of the clitoris. Though some trauma survivors I know rave about this experience, I didn't feel safe during the workshop I tried (with Kurt). It made me aware that there are many workshops and experiences marketed to individuals in search of sexual healing. Do your research and trust your gut about what is right for *you*.

20. **Sexological Bodywork (via hands-on Tantra session)**

Sexological Bodywork is a kind of hands-on erotic education. My tantra sessions—though not technically Sexological Bodywork—were close enough to give you an idea of what could go on in a session like this. Sessions might include breath work, sensual massage, erotic instruction, touch, or other modalities. I was helped by this kind of work, but you'll want to find a reputable practitioner. If you're interested, check out *sexologicalbodyworkers.org* or *somaticinstitute.com*.

21. **Eye Movement Desensitization and Reprocessing (EMDR)**

EMDR is frequently used for a variety of trauma, and there is strong evidence of its efficacy. In essence, EMDR is designed to help a person regulate emotions (or traumatic stress) related to traumatic memories or experiences. In my case, I didn't continue with this modality because it didn't directly address my sex problems. I would try it again, however, if a situation called for it. I always felt great after these sessions. Very empowered.

22. **Betty Dodson's Bodysex Workshops**

I covered most of my Betty Dodson experience in Chapter 16. I'll add here that Betty and Carlin's website is a treasure trove of sex ed. See the Recommended Resources section. And Betty is still doing her Bodysex weekends!

23. **Dildos**

Dildos are sex toys designed for insertion. They can be very beneficial in preventing narrowing of the vagina due to GSM. If you're single and over forty, you might want to invest in one, even if you already have a vibrator. If pelvic rehabilitation involves penetration (like dilator use), ask your doctor or therapist if you can use a dildo in coordination—possibly not at first, but eventually. This can help make recovery more erotic.

24. **Vibrators**

These sex toys provide stimulation through vibration. Vibrators can be a fab way to reconnect to your sexuality—solo or with a partner. See my website for different options. Also, ask your PT or doctor if vibration can be used in conjunction with other therapies. Restoring sexual pleasure might need this bit of fun.

25. **Sensate Focus**

I didn't have room in this story to go into more detail about Sensate Focus. I wish I did because this technique, which exists in many forms, is often transformative for couples (and individuals) finding their way back to sensual connection. Originally developed by Masters and Johnson, this technique is shared by many online. Sensate Focus is very often used as part of sex therapy.

26. **Hormone Replacement Therapy (HRT)**

See my website for extended information about combatting dryness, especially in conjunction with GSM.

27. **Vaginal Moisturizers**

I included moisturizers since finding one I liked was a mini-adventure in itself. See my website for extended information about GSM.

28. **Healing Habits / The Pleasure Hour**

See the section on How to Create Your Own Pleasure Hour.

29. **Lingerie**

Under this category, I'll include anything that makes you feel great and turns you on. Try saving your best pieces for your own eyes.

30. **Self-Study**

Books played a significant role in shaping my thinking throughout my whole process. There's so much information out there. With a library card, there's no telling what kind of help you can get for free.

And Now, a Little Anatomy

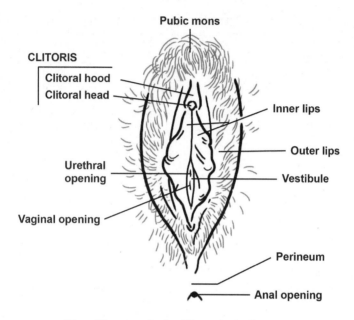

View of the external vulva. Illustration by Simone Nemes.

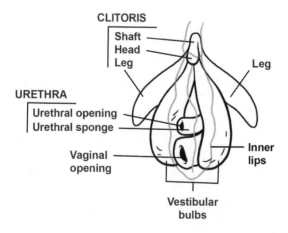

View of the internal clitoris. Illustration by Simone Nemes.

Solving Common
(and Uncommon) Sex Problems

Please refer to *LauraZam.com* for the latest research regarding libido, arousal, orgasm, pelvic pain, genital skin changes, endometriosis, and more.

About Genitourinary Syndrome
of Menopause (GSM)

GSM is a relatively new terminology replacing "atrophy," and it's a good move by the medical community because it covers a broader swath of symptoms. Unfortunately, too many women approaching perimenopause and menopause are blindsided by the different ways low hormones can adversely affect their genitals and sex life.

Symptoms include decreased lubrication, increased propensity for bacterial and yeast infections, painful intercourse, narrowing and shortening of the vagina, loss of labia minora (inner lips), thinning of vaginal tissue, burning inside the canal, soreness at the vaginal opening (in the vestibule), inflammation of tissue surrounding urethra (G-spot area), vaginismus, pelvic pain, inflammation of vulvar tissue (vaginitis), and bleeding during sex. *I know, right?*

Please don't freak out by how many things can go wrong. Not everyone will have all these problems. And, even if you *are* affected, available remedies have a great track record for helping those with GSM. The goal is to find what's best for you. For that reason, I've compiled a comprehensive, constantly updated list of treatments on my website. All medical information has been compiled with the input of Rachel S. Rubin, MD, a nationally recognized urologic surgeon and sexual medicine specialist in Washington, DC.

One more thing about GSM: when you go to the doctor for symptoms (and I hope you do seek medical treatment), your physician may prescribe what this physician prefers—without giving you a full overview of options! It's best to get educated about your choices before seeing your doc. Check my website for these options.

How to Find a Sexual Healing Expert

It's critical to find a key practitioner who is *very* knowledgeable when it comes to human sexuality—and your problem in particular. Unfortunately, standard training programs for physicians, therapists, and other providers include little (if any) sex education. Plenty of experts exist, though, and there are many avenues for finding them. Additional experts, including individual practitioners, can be found on my website.

Menopause Specialist (Doctors and Other Practitioners):
- North American Menopause Society (NAMS), *Menopause.org*

Pelvic Pain Specialist (Doctors and Other Practitioners):
- National Vulvodynia Association (NVA), *NVA.org*

Sexual Medicine Specialist (Doctors and Other Practitioners):
- International Society for the Study of Women's Sexual Health (ISSWSH), *ISSWSH.org*

Pelvic Floor Physical Therapist:
- National Vulvodynia Association (NVA), *NVA.org*

Sex Therapist:
- American Association for Sexuality Educators, Counselors and Therapists (AASECT), *aasect.org*. Please note: though many therapists say they practice "sex therapy," not all of

them have gone through a rigorous AASECT certification program. If possible, choose a sex therapist with this certification (found via the AASECT website).

Sex Counselor:

- American Association for Sexuality Educators, Counselors and Therapists (AASECT), *aasect.org*. Sex Counselors are people with counseling certification who have gone through special training in human sexuality. Again, best to stick with those certified through AASECT.

Sexuality Educator:

- American Association for Sexuality Educators, Counselors and Therapists (AASECT), *aasect.org*. Freelance sexuality educators do exist, though, anyone can call themselves a sex educator or sexologist. AASECT, again, is your friend here in finding a qualified educator. If trauma or medical concerns are a culprit, then you might want to make sure you see a therapist and/or physician as well. Please note: some sexuality educators also have other degrees. A doctor could also be certified as a sex educator, for instance. Once again, *aasect.org* is your best resource.
- Adult stores. Adult stores, good ones, are often staffed with sexuality educators. To find a shop that has this expertise, search for shops in your area, scrutinizing their websites.

Sexual Healing Coach:

- American Association for Sexuality Educators, Counselors and Therapists (AASECT), *aasect.org*. Some sexuality educators, counselors, and therapists also do coaching. Again, check out the AASECT website. Coaching will be more active than an educational experience, but it's not therapy. Coaching should not be in lieu of therapy or medical care if complex psychological issues or medical issues are present.

- Somatica Institute, *Somaticainstitute.com*. This organization has a good reputation, though I've not tried them myself. They certify coaches that work through talk and also touch.

Books Mentioned in *The Pleasure Plan*

Berman, Laura. *Loving Sex: The Book of Joy and Passion*. New York, NY: DK, 2011.

Perel, Esther. *Mating in Captivity: Unlocking Erotic Intelligence*. New York, NY: HarperCollins, 2006.

Nagoski, Emily. *Come as You Are: The Surprising New Science That Will Transform Your Sex Life*. New York, NY: Simon & Schuster, 2015.

Jong, Erica. *Fear of Flying*. New York, NY: New American Library, 1973.

Jethá, Cacilda, and Christopher Ryan. *Sex at Dawn: How We Mate, Why We Stray, and What It Means for Modern Relationships*. New York, NY: Harper Perennial, 2011.

Hollander, Xaviera. *The Happy Hooker's Guide to Sex: 69 Orgasmic Ways to Pleasure a Woman*. New York, NY: Skyhorse Publishing, 2008.

For a list of additional books on sexual healing, visit *LauraZam.com*.

Recommended Resources

This list is constantly being updated. For the most up-to-date information, check out my website, *LauraZam.com*. I also send around my newest finds via my *Zam Not Spam* newsletter.

General Sex Ed

- Betty Dodson's website, *DodsonandRoss.com*. This is the sex-ed site run by Betty Dodson and Carlin Ross. It's very comprehensive and informative.
- Institute for Sexuality Education and Enlightenment (ISEE), *Instituteforsexuality.com*. This Institute offers affordable, terrific courses on all areas of sex ed. This is my sex-ed school.

Sexual Exploration

- XConfessions, *Xconfessions.com*. An ethical video porn site with a female gaze.
- FetLife, *Fetlife.com*. A good place to start if you're interested in exploring BDSM, fetish, or kink.
- Literotica, *Literotica.com*. A site that features erotic stories.
- Dipsea, *Dipseastories.com*. A new app of erotic stories.
- Urban Tantra site, *BarbaraCarellas.com*. A great place to begin an exploration of tantra.

Sexual Problems and Solutions

- *LauraZam.com*. I'm constantly finding new solutions for sexual issues. Best to check out my website for the latest.

Trauma Recovery

- Bessel van der Kolk's site, *Besselvanderkolk.net*. Dr. van der Kolk is a preeminent thinker, doctor, and voice in the trauma community.

- Rape, Abuse & Incest National Network (RAINN), *RAINN.org*. This organization plays a crucial role in helping prevent sexual crimes, and healing in the aftermath. Their website is chock full of important resources.
- Darkness to Light, *D2L.org*. A site for people who were sexually abused as children, or those who are interested in prevention and advocacy around this issue. Many terrific resources.

Relationships

- Esther Perel's website, *Estherperel.com*. This site offers wonderful resources and wisdom for individuals and couples. Perel also has a few must-read books.
- Intimacy Retreats, *Intimacyretreats.com*. This is the great retreat featured in my book.
- Imago Relationship, *Harvilleandhelen.com*. This couple has a unique model for helping couples grow their relationship. Highly recommended.

Time Management

- Pomodoro website, *FrancescoCerillo.com*. In my opinion, ongoing healing habits go hand-in-hand with good time management. I swear by this technique.

How to Create Your Own Pleasure Hour

On the surface, a *Pleasure Hour* is really simple: sixty minutes of good feelings, once a week. The tricky part is keeping this appointment with yourself. The tips below, for the most part, pertain to maintaining your hour.

1. Set a time you can stick with every week.

2. If you don't have a full hour on any given week, use the time you have—even if it's ten minutes.

3. If your regularly scheduled time is not possible due to an unforeseen event, feel free to reschedule for that week. Try to keep some dedicated time with yourself, no matter what.

4. If you miss a week (or more), it doesn't matter. Just move forward with an appointment.

5. At your session, you can think of this dedicated time any way you'd like. Here are some ideas: take a bath, experiment with your vibrator, go for a walk, do Kegels, watch porn, read a book or magazine, pet your dog, eat berries, stroke your skin, work with dilators, take a nap. If you don't feel like engaging sexually for your hour, that's fine. Just ask yourself: What would be pleasurable right now? Let pleasure tell you what you need to find wholeness. Pleasure might just be your healer.

How to Host Your Own Sex Brunch

You can hold a Sex Brunch as a formal gathering, as a fun activity to do with a group of friends, as part of another event, in combination with a book club, or in another setting where you'd like to encourage folks to talk about sex. Below are some very general guidelines.

1. **Create Your Attendee List**

   Choose a group of people that might benefit from this gathering. One gender? Mixed? A particular age range? It's up to you.

2. **Decide on Logistics**

   Some considerations are obvious, like where and for how long. But be creative in crafting an event that works for you and your group. In addition to the Sex Brunch in my book, I've held these events in libraries, bookstores, and even the lobby of my building. I've had conversation only events, and also gatherings where I invited an expert to present (like a sex toy aficionado). I've fully hosted and also have done these as potlucks. In some instances, I had everyone read a book beforehand (see below).

3. **Create a Safe Space**

At the Brunch, start with ground rules. Elicit these by asking the group what they need to feel safe, capturing their requirements on chart paper or a whiteboard. Make sure you post their responses somewhere in the room.

4. **Use Index Cards**

In this way, attendees can write questions anonymously.

5. **Let the Conversation Flow**

I mean, allow it to organically evolve. If there's a lull, read an index card. If people seem more interested in speaking spontaneously, let them. Try not to control it too much. Enjoy!

To get a FREE Sex Brunch kit, visit *LauraZam.com/SexBrunch*.

Using *The Pleasure Plan* Book for Your Sex Brunch

A terrific way to help attendees feel comfortable sharing and asking questions is to have them read *The Pleasure Plan* beforehand. See the following page for question ideas.

Reading Group and Sex Brunch Questions

1. In *The Pleasure Plan*, Laura tells a story, from her twenties, about wanting to be sexy versus wanting to have sex. She explores how these desires intersect throughout the book. What is your understanding of sexiness? What is your understanding of sexual desire?

2. In Chapter 9, Laura visits the house where she was sexually abused as a four-year-old. Was this a wise move? Have you ever done anything daring, or unusual, to face your own demons?

3. In Chapter 10, Laura sees a trauma therapist who tells her that as long as she has agency (a sense of personal empowerment) she doesn't have any significant trauma residue. Do you agree with this assessment?

4. In Chapter 17, Laura learns that she has vaginal atrophy. Is atrophy (or GSM) something you were aware of? Is it an issue you speak about with your friends, family, or others in your circle?

5. Laura's mother plays a crucial role in this book. Would you have enjoyed having a mom like Harriet, Laura's mom? Why? Why not?

6. Laura explores two naked treatments toward the end of the book: a private Tantra session and Betty Dodson's Body-sex workshop. Did you find these adventures intriguing? Extreme? Could you see yourself doing something similar? Why? Why not?

7. In Chapter 19, Laura invites her sexual problems into bed with her, in order to understand what they all require. Do you think

this was a wise move? Could you see yourself doing something similar?

8. Laura takes a circuitous route to healing and does not always follow through with treatments. Did you find this frustrating at times? If you were her friend, what would you have said to her during this journey?

9. Which curative adventure do you think helped Laura the most, in terms of healing? What about in terms of her relationship?

10. What is your biggest take away from *The Pleasure Plan*?

About the Author

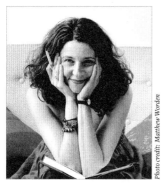

Photo credit: Matthew Worden

Laura Zam is a Sexuality Educator, Certified Trauma Professional, award-winning solo performer, *HuffPost* blogger, TEDx speaker, and workshop leader, whose work focuses on sexual healing.

Her writing appears in the *New York Times* (Modern Love), *Salon*, *HuffPost*, *SheKnows*, *NextTribe*, *The Forward*, in international journals, and in five book anthologies.

She lives in Washington, DC, with her husband and too many throw pillows. Visit: *www.laurazam.com*.